The Secrets *of* Living *and* Loving *with* Diabetes

Three Experts Answer Questions You've Always Wanted to Ask

Janis Roszler, RD, CDE, LD/N

William H. Polonsky, PhD, CDE

Steven V. Edelman, MD

S

SURREY BOOKS

Chicago

The Secrets of Living and Loving with Diabetes is published by
Surrey Books, Inc., 230 E. Ohio St., Suite 120, Chicago, IL 60611

First edition: 1 2 3 4 5

This book is manufactured in the United States of America

Library of Congress Cataloging-in-Publication data:

Roszler, Janis.
    The secrets of living and loving with diabetes : three experts answer
questions you've always wanted to ask / Janis Roszler, William H. Polonsky,
Steven V. Edelman.— 1st ed.
       p. cm.
    ISBN 1-57284-066-8
    1. Diabetes—Popular works. I. Polonsky, William H., 1952- II. Edelman,
Steven V. III. Title.

RC660.4.R689 2004
616.4'62—dc22   2004020933

Editorial services: Bookcrafters, Inc., Chicago
Cover design: Joan Sommers Design, Chicago

For prices on quantity purchases, contact Surrey Books at:
www.surreybooks.com

This title is distributed to the trade by Publishers Group West

Disclaimers

Praise from Diabetes Experts

"This book will help anyone with diabetes learn to live a better and happier life."
—Jay S. Skyler, MD, Past President, American Diabetes Association

"An outstanding book, written by an exceptional team."
—Lance Porter, Editor-in-Chief, *Diabetes Positive*

"A commonsense approach to an often overwhelming disease."
—Joan Hill, RD, CDE, LD, American Dietetic Assoc. Educator of the Year, Joslin Diabetes Center

"This book goes beyond—way beyond—the meat and potatoes of diabetes care. It gives you answers and insights to the endless quandaries of balancing real life with the distresses and strains of dealing with diabetes."
—Hope S. Warshaw, MMSc, RD, CDE, author of *Eat Out, Eat Right!*

"It's like having a unique and wonderful support group in a book."
—Itamar Raz, MD, President, Israel Diabetes Assoc.

"Filled with real life experiences, this book covers issues that were only discussed behind closed doors. It's the one book that answers all your questions about dealing with diabetes in social situations and personal relationships."
—Audrey Finklestein, Executive Vice President, Animas Corp.

This book is dedicated to:

My loving husband, Myer, and my cool kids, Elisheva, Shira, Rachel, and Amichai.

—Janis

Wonderful Reegan, the love of my life.

—Bill

Ingrid, my super wife, and my beautiful daughters, Talia and Carina.

—Steve

Acknowledgments

We thank our patients and friends who shared their personal stories, and the members of the Diabetes Care and Education (DCE) practice group of the American Dietetic Association for their comments and story contributions. Most of all, we thank our families, friends, and colleagues for their support; Susan Schwartz, our publisher, and Hope Warshaw for their enthusiasm about this project; Corky Kessler for his invaluable guidance; Harvey Cohn and Veta "Joy" Reid for their critical eyes; and Lisa Bauch for her editing wizardry.

Contents

Foreword

Having diabetes is a challenge 24/7. It's a challenge that doesn't go away. Accepting that challenge—truly accepting it—is what *The Secrets of Living and Loving with Diabetes* is all about. This book recognizes and appreciates the fact that having diabetes impacts all aspects of one's life, all the time. It also recognizes the reciprocal: that everything in life has an impact on diabetes and how one lives with it.

The authors have taken a very friendly, warm, sensitive, and quite knowledgeable approach in this book. It is written not just for people with diabetes; it also gives equal importance to those who live with or love someone with diabetes. It recognizes that there are many more people affected by diabetes than the number who actually have the disease.

Using straight talk and personalized stories, this book provides practical advice—for both those with diabetes and their loved ones—on how to handle common situations that arise every day. In that sense, it truly provides insight into living with diabetes. The book also describes how to enlist support, both emotional and hands-on, from family and friends.

Most chapters conclude with a section on what the person with diabetes wants loved ones to know and, conversely, what loved ones want the person with diabetes to know. Throughout, you are encouraged to examine your motivations and express your feelings in the interest of smoother interpersonal relationships and the development of

positive attitudes that often contribute to successful out-
comes. The book accomplishes its objectives with simple
practical examples and straightforward advice.

An especially helpful feature of *The Secrets of Living and
Loving with Diabetes* are the specific exercises found in most
chapters that involve readers in quizzes, questions, checklists,
and coping strategies. Often, the person with diabetes as well
as their loved one are invited to participate in the activities
and then compare answers. This encourages true communication and understanding of important issues, feelings, ideas,
and concerns.

This book is to be read, absorbed, and lived. It is a
real primer that will help anyone with diabetes—or affected
by another's diabetes—learn to live a better and happier life.

Jay S. Skyler, MD
Past President, American Diabetes Association;
Professor of Medicine, Pediatrics, and Psychology,
Division of Endocrinology, Diabetes & Metabolism,
University of Miami, Florida

Introduction

When you look out into a waiting room and see someone crying, you can't help but be moved.

Life can be challenging for people with diabetes and their loved ones. Too often, it is made more difficult because of misunderstandings or a lack of reliable information. Diabetes shouldn't sabotage anyone's relationships. That is why we wrote this book.

The Secrets of Living and Loving with Diabetes is designed to help individuals minimize the negative effects that diabetes can have on their relationships. In it, we examine many questions that don't always receive clear answers, such as:

1. How can I keep diabetes from dominating my relationships?

2. What can I do about relatives who nag me about my diabetes?

3. How can I motivate a loved one who ignores his or her diabetes?

4. How can I become more motivated about my diabetes control?

5. What should I do in an emergency? When is a problem a true emergency?

6. What do blood sugar test results mean? How can I use them to improve my control?

7. Whom should I tell about my diabetes? How do I tell them? What if they don't understand? What if my boss doesn't understand?

8. What is diabetes etiquette? Is there a right way and a wrong way to tend to diabetes needs in public?

9. How can I keep diabetes concerns out of the bedroom?

If you have diabetes or care about someone who has it, this book is for you. *The Secrets of Living and Loving with Diabetes* is filled with expert advice, quizzes, discussion topics, suggested activities, and personal stories.

How to Use This Book

Read this book alone or with someone you love. Start with the first chapter so that you and your partner share an accurate definition of diabetes. Then enjoy the remaining chapters in any order. Participate together in the assorted discussion topics and quizzes. They are there to prompt conversation, help resolve pressing issues, and hopefully prevent new problems from developing.

Each chapter ends with a quick list of concerns that you may wish to share about the topics presented. This list is certainly not complete. You may have additional feelings and ideas that you wish to communicate after reading these chapters. Don't hesitate. Voice your needs and concerns so others can offer their support and help.

We have made every effort to write this book in common language that can be easily understood by all. Medical terms are clearly defined. We've used the terms "blood glucose" and "blood sugar" interchangeably, just as our patients do. Blood glucose values are provided in mg/dl, the form used in the U.S., and in mmol/L, which is typically used throughout the world. If you have issues that are not included in this book, please share them with us.

E-mail your comments to: dearjanis@yahoo.com.

Chapter One

Hey, Who Invited You?

If you have diabetes or love someone who has diabetes, you know that it comes along on every outing, shows up at every meal, and follows you wherever you go—even into the bedroom at night. How well do you know this uninvited intruder?

> "Do you know what diabetes is?" asked the diabetes educator
>
> "Sure," answered Ella. "I've had it for 15 years. I have sugar in my blood, lots of it. I just have to stay away from eating sugar. I don't let my family eat it, either. You should hear me yell when I see my kids walk into the house with a candy bar. I'm not going to let them get diabetes, and I know if they keep eating those candy bars, they will!"

Many types of diabetes exist and, dear Ella, none comes from eating a candy bar. The most common forms are type 1, type 2, and gestational. Each has a different cause and initial appearance, but all lead to high blood sugar and other changes that can wreak enormous damage if left untreated. Fortunately, good medical care can help you avoid serious problems and live a long, healthy life with diabetes. Regardless of the type of diabetes, many of the basic treatment strategies are the same: regular physical activity, a healthy meal plan, blood glucose monitoring, and medication.

Type 1 Diabetes

Formerly called juvenile-onset or insulin-dependent diabetes, this form of diabetes can start at any time but usually appears before age 30. It is caused by the destruction of the body's insulin-producing cells, called beta cells, located in the pancreas. This cell breakdown is due to an autoimmune response, which means that, for reasons not yet known, the body labels these beneficial beta cells as "the enemy" and tries to kill them.

As beta cells are destroyed, the body loses its ability to produce insulin, a hormone needed to utilize the energy that comes from food. Great amounts of the foods we eat are transformed into glucose (sugar), which is the main fuel source for our bodies, and insulin allows the glucose in the blood to enter the cells of the body. Without insulin, you can't absorb most of the energy from food. And without insulin, the sugar in your bloodstream reaches higher and higher levels, which, over an extended period of time (months to years), can lead to damage to the organs of the body such as eyes, kidneys, nerves, and blood vessels.

Prior to the discovery of insulin in 1922, death was a common outcome of diabetes. Thanks to insulin and other technological advances, it is possible to live a long and healthy life with type 1 diabetes. But people with type 1 must take outside sources of insulin to make up for their missing beta cells and keep their bodies functioning properly. Approximately 5–10 percent of people with diabetes have type 1.

When I learned that I had type 1 diabetes, I was stunned; it came on so suddenly. I was 18 and had all of the classic symptoms—weight loss, excessive thirst, frequent urination, fatigue, incredible hunger, and wounds that wouldn't heal. I remember drinking and drinking and never having my thirst quenched. What an odd sensation! My friends couldn't stand my frequent trips to the bathroom and didn't want to invite me anywhere. Imagine walking through the mall and having to run to the bathroom time and time again. Even my family was impatient with me. Finding out that I had diabetes came as a relief to everyone, including me. With treatment, my symptoms improved immediately, my friends and family offered amazing support, and I got my life back.

—Katie

Type 2 Diabetes

Unlike people with type 1 diabetes, individuals with type 2 diabetes, formerly called adult-onset, or non-insulin-dependent diabetes, produce insulin (at least in the early stages of the disease), but their bodies are unable to use it. This is known as "insulin resistance." Just as in type 1, this problem can lead to excessive levels of sugar in the bloodstream. Without proper treatment the sugar levels in your bloodstream will climb too high. Chronic elevation of these levels over months and years can lead to damage of important organs such as the kidneys, nerves, eyes, and blood vessels.

Heredity plays a large part in determining who might develop type 2 diabetes, but obesity and inactivity also play significant roles. Type 2 usually appears after age 30, but it can occur earlier. Sadly, skyrocketing rates of obesity in young people have led to an epidemic number of children with type 2. About 90 percent of all people with diabetes have type 2.

I couldn't believe it when the doctor said I had diabetes. I am 63 years old and knew that I had gained a lot of weight, but I felt great. I had no symptoms at all—no blurred vision or tingling in the feet that I had heard about. My wife, Rhonda, and I had so much to learn. She needed to know which foods to buy and how to prepare them, and I had to learn about my body and my new needs. We took this on as a family learning project. We all started living healthier.

—Morris

Gestational Diabetes

This is the "pregnancy" type of diabetes, and it occurs in approximately 7 percent of all pregnant women. As in type 2, the body becomes insulin resistant, leading to increasingly higher blood sugar levels. The most likely trigger for gestational diabetes is the hormonal changes that take place in a woman's body during pregnancy. Without treatment, the baby's health is also at risk. In addition, the mother may have a more difficult delivery since a fetus in this type of pregnancy tends to gain more weight.

Proper treatment may involve diet, exercise, and sometimes medication throughout the pregnancy. Gestational diabetes is not passed on to the baby, but it does put the mother at higher risk of developing type 2 diabetes in the future. About 25 percent of women who have gestational diabetes will eventually develop type 2.

Janis, one of our authors, shares her personal story:

I didn't fit any of the textbook profiles. As a registered dietitian and certified diabetes educator, I always exercised regularly, maintained a proper weight, and ate healthfully. My diagnosis came as a big surprise. I had taught diabetes care for more than 10 years when I was diagnosed, but until that time had only "talked the talk," and never "walked the walk."

One doesn't have to have diabetes to understand how to deal with it, but having it made a huge impact on me. I had to stick to a special meal plan and watch the clock like a hawk so that my blood sugar checks would be at exactly the right time. Diabetes took over my life and the lives of everyone in my family. My kids carried my glucose monitor and test strips. My husband overlooked my pregnancy moods that were made even crazier because of my blood sugar swings, poor guy.

Type 1, type 2, and gestational diabetes are becoming increasingly "popular." Americans are in the grips of a diabetes epidemic, with the numbers of people affected growing larger every day. According to the American Diabetes Association, 18.2 million people in the United States, over 6 percent of the population, have diabetes. Around 13 million have been diagnosed and about 5.2 million don't know that they have the disease. Worldwide, more than 194 million people have diabetes. By the year 2030, experts say that over 370 million people will be diabetic. Estimates indicate that 1 out of every 3 Americans born in 2000 will get diabetes.

When Definitions Differ

Sally and Bill are at odds with each other, which is a problem since they are engaged to be married in a few months. "It's like he's trying to kill himself," Sally laments. "When I say anything, he just gets angry with me." Sally is convinced that Bill's big problem is the cookies, candy, and other sweets that he eats. Yet Bill takes his medications, checks his blood sugar regularly, and has started walking every day. In fact, Bill's recent blood tests revealed that his average blood sugars are in an excellent range. As far as he can tell, eating sweets hasn't hurt him at all, but Sally's constant nagging has.

You can't manage diabetes effectively if you don't have all the facts. Do you and your loved ones know enough about diabetes? Some of the biggest family arguments about diabetes occur when individuals and family members hold different or inaccurate beliefs.

Let's find out what you and the person most likely to be supporting your effort to manage diabetes really know, and who knows more. Take this true/false quiz separately from your partner or loved one. Each of you can write your answers, "True" or "False," on separate sheets of paper.

Then check them against the correct answers—and explanations—that follow the quiz.

1. Type 1 diabetes is much more serious than type 2.
   True or False?

2. After you have had diabetes for many years, complications like eye, nerve, and kidney disease are inevitable.
   True or False?

3. Eating lots of sugary food is the major cause of diabetes.
   True or False?

4. The most important method for controlling diabetes is to avoid foods that contain sugar.
   True or False?

5. People with good family support are more likely to be successful in managing their diabetes.
   True or False?

6. The time to start worrying about controlling your diabetes is when you first develop complications or other bothersome symptoms.
   True or False?

7. Carefully following a healthy meal plan is all you need to do to manage your diabetes.
   True or False?

8. If you feel well, your diabetes is probably under control.
   True or False?

9. If you have type 2 diabetes and the doctor prescribes insulin, you haven't adequately taken care of your diabetes.
   True or False?

10. Controlling your blood sugar is the only key to a long and healthy life.
    True or False?

To find out how well each of you did, let's examine these topics one by one and separate fact from fiction.

1. Type 1 diabetes is much more serious than type 2. FALSE

> A few years ago, I developed type 2 diabetes. I was so relieved to learn that I didn't have real diabetes. I mean, it isn't real if I don't have to take insulin, right? I started exercising, and luckily my blood sugars improved. Now I'm cured. I don't test my blood anymore and certainly don't tell anyone that I had diabetes. I'm out of danger; at least I think I am.
>
> —Mark

A misunderstanding among many people is that type 2 diabetes is less serious than type 1. The fact is that diabetes is serious no matter what type you have. And it is *real* diabetes, regardless of the way you control it. Type 1 and type 2 may differ in how they develop in the body, but if left untreated, both will lead to devastating complications such as heart attack and stroke, sexual dysfunction, nerve damage, kidney failure, blindness, amputation, and even death. Possible cures such as cell implants are being researched but are not available yet.

If your symptoms disappear, that doesn't mean you are cured, just that you may be doing a terrific job of controlling your diabetes. If you are keeping your A1C level (measure of blood glucose control over the past two to three months), your blood pressure, and your cholesterol level in great shape, you should be extremely proud of yourself.

2. After you have had diabetes for many years, complications like eye, nerve, and kidney disease are inevitable. FALSE

> My aunt Katherine lost her leg to diabetes when she was 63 years old. My cousin Larry lost his eyesight from it and

had to use a guide dog. Both took horrible care of themselves, really horrible. They ignored everything that they were told to do, missed doctors' appointments, and ate junk. I think they wanted it to turn out the way it did.

—Dina

Diabetes is not a death sentence and complications are not inevitable. When you say the word "diabetes," scary images of amputation, blindness, and kidney dialysis come to mind. Most families have friends or relatives who have had serious complications. While you may be familiar with these disturbing stories, you may not have heard enough good stories. Many people live for years with diabetes and develop few or no complications. Is this just luck? Well, genetic differences do play a role, but the biggest factor is good diabetes care.

Two impressive research studies, the nationwide Diabetes Control and Complications Trial (DCCT) and the United Kingdom Prospective Diabetes Study (UKPDS), demonstrated the importance of good diabetes control in helping people avoid complications. The DCCT showed that individuals with type 1 could lower their risk of complications by up to 50 percent if they maintained their blood sugar (glucose) in as normal a range as possible. The UKPDS reported similar results for those with type 2. Relax. With today's medical advances, you can almost always avoid serious complications.

3. Eating lots of sugary food is the major cause of diabetes. FALSE

A "sweet tooth" does not cause diabetes, but that doesn't mean you should drop this book and run out to the candy section of your local grocery store. The two major contributors to type 1 diabetes are heredity and certain environmental factors not yet clearly understood by researchers. In type 2, genetics plays a very large role. Lifestyle, obesity, and age also play a part in developing diabetes, but you won't get type 2 unless you have inherited the potential to develop this condition. Don't blame yourself and don't blame others with diabetes. It is not their fault.

4. The most important method for controlling diabetes is to avoid foods that contain sugar. FALSE

Let's revisit our friends Sally and Bill. Was Sally right to insist that Bill eliminate cookies, candy, and other desserts from his diet? Perhaps in the past, medical professionals would have complemented her vigilance. Not today. If Bill's A1C level (his average measure of blood sugar levels for the past two to three months; see Chapter 5) is fine and his blood pressure and cholesterol levels are good, then there is no problem in eating reasonable amounts of the foods he likes. But even if levels are not ideal, dietary recommendations are now flexible and allow for foods that everyone loves. Even alcohol has a place in most diabetes meal plans.

Today's regimens are all about promoting good health and a positive quality of life. If you desire a particular food, a registered dietitian who specializes in diabetes will usually find a way to fit it into a well-balanced meal plan. Sally and Bill, don't let food misunderstandings strain your relationship. Meet with a dietitian or read through current diabetes publications to get the facts.

5. People with good family support are more likely to be successful managing their diabetes. TRUE

Don't underestimate the power of a loving family. German researchers recently asked 59 patients with type 2 diabetes to invite their spouses to accompany them to diabetes class. The study, published in December, 2003, found that spouse participation actually helped patients improve their blood glucose control. The support of family and friends makes a tremendous difference in a person's diabetes control and quality of life. Remember, diabetes doesn't only affect the people who have it, it also affects everyone around them.

Here are some suggestions on how you can support a spouse, family member, or friend who has diabetes:

a. Attend diabetes class together

b. Share diabetes publications

c. Read this book

d. Provide diabetes newsletters to friends and coworkers who show an interest in learning more

e. Exercise together

f. Spend time together and discuss issues that are troubling

g. Eat together. Food choices recommended for a diabetes meal plan are healthy for the entire family

Participate in community diabetes advocacy and fundraising programs, such as walk-a-thons and bike-a-thons. Contact the American Diabetes Association at www.diabetes.org or call 1-800-DIABETES to find out about upcoming events in your area.

6. The time to start worrying about controlling your diabetes is when you first develop complications or other bothersome symptoms. FALSE

The best time to focus on your diabetes is now. Don't wait. If you don't have diabetic complications, take steps to prevent them before they appear. If challenging symptoms such as vision problems or pain and tingling in your feet have already made an appearance, you can still stop these problems from getting worse. Don't stress out about diabetes.

Learn what you can do to achieve the best health possible and enlist everyone's support.

7. Carefully following a healthy meal plan is all you need to do to manage your diabetes. FALSE

Following a healthy diabetes meal plan is just one of the many methods to manage diabetes. If you eat well but don't take your medication, participate in regular physical activity, or monitor your blood glucose, cholesterol, and blood pressure, achieving good diabetes control will be a challenge. Physical activity is a terrific way to maintain a healthy weight, normalize blood sugar levels, and trigger hormones that can improve your mood.

8. If you feel well, your diabetes is probably under control. FALSE

If only that were true! Unfortunately, people with diabetes do not always experience symptoms. You may feel terrific even when your blood sugar and blood pressure are out of control. When glucose levels have been high for a long time, your body may acclimate to that elevated level and feel normal. A subsequent decrease to a healthy range can initially feel uncomfortably low. Many people believe that they know exactly what their blood sugar is without checking; research shows, however, that most blood sugar guesses are incorrect.

Most people cannot tell if their blood pressure is too high. This is similar to high cholesterol, which has no symptoms, either. Elevated blood pressure over time significantly increases the risk for stroke, which occurs two to four times more often in people with diabetes. The majority of people with diabetes have blood pressure high enough to warrant treatment, which can be very effective. Don't make important decisions based on how you feel. Check the numbers and go from there.

9. If you have type 2 diabetes and the doctor prescribes insulin, you haven't adequately taken care of your diabetes. FALSE

> I was so terrified of needles. I am 58 and have had type 2 diabetes for about 15 years. I swore to myself that I would never take insulin. First my physician, Dr. Rogers, used the prospect of insulin as leverage. He hinted that if I didn't take care of my diabetes, I would have to use it. Sound like a punishment? I thought so, too. So when he finally told me it was time to begin insulin, I was sure that I had failed. I could see the same reaction in my husband Vincent's face. He thought that I had failed too. On the ride home from the doctor's office, he accused me of neglecting my diabetes and putting myself and my life at risk. "See, you finally did it!" he said.
>
> —Doris

Have you failed if you need to begin insulin injections? Absolutely not! Insulin used to be prescribed only for people with type 1 diabetes. Now we know that individuals with type 2 can also benefit greatly from the additional control insulin offers. In fact, close to half of all Americans with type 2 take insulin. Diabetes can be harder to manage over time, and the need for insulin is often a natural development of the disease.

Is it an emotional challenge to face the fact that you need to give yourself injections each day? Yes, it can be. Many people delay starting the insulin treatment because they are afraid. The truth is that once people try insulin, they feel so much better that they kick themselves for not starting therapy sooner. Don't deny yourself, or the ones you love, this important treatment. Portable insulin-containing "pens," smaller needles, and improved insulin make these options excellent and comfortable choices.

10. Controlling your blood sugar is the only key to a long and healthy life. FALSE

Keeping your blood sugar level as normal as possible is essential, but this is only one of the important keys to successful diabetes management. Two out of three people with diabetes die from heart disease or stroke, making maintaining normal blood pressure and cholesterol levels a priority. Elevated blood pressure can damage your kidneys. And if the body's level of artery-clogging cholesterol (called LDL cholesterol) is too high, blood vessels will narrow and put stress on the heart as it tries to circulate the blood.

A long and healthy life is a realistic goal with diabetes. Exercise, diet, and medication all help this goal become a reality. With diabetes, controlling blood pressure is just as important as controlling blood sugar.

So, how did you do? Compare your answers with your partner's. Who scored highest? Before you complete this chapter, take time to discuss what you both learned from this brief exercise:

1. How did your answers differ?

2. Where did you both agree?

3. Did any of the information surprise you?

4. What did you both learn?

Diabetes is a complex topic. Take the time to learn all you can about it. The following are suggestions to help guide you.

Create a Home Diabetes Library

Develop your own personal reference library (and read it!). Acquire books published by nationally recognized and respected diabetes experts and organizations such as the American Diabetes Association, Joslin Diabetes Center at Harvard University, International Diabetes Center, TCOYD (Taking Control of Your Diabetes), and the Diabetes Research Institute. You'll find information on how to contact these organizations in Suggested Resources at the back of this book.

Approaches continue to change. Meal planning is much more flexible than it was in the past, and new treatments are constantly being developed. If you have older books in your library, replace them with newer publications. Visit your local bookseller with a friend and browse through the shelves. Enjoy the immense variety of available books on diabetes. To make certain that you choose well, keep in mind the following:

1. Search for books that are written by respected authors who are affiliated with recognized diabetes organizations, such as those listed above.

2. Purchase current titles. Diabetes treatments keep changing. Pass by the used book shops.

3. Buy a basic guide to diabetes for your collection, but consider purchasing other books as well. Thousands of excellent books are available on topics that include meal planning, exercise, the emotional side of diabetes, and even insulin pumps. See Suggested References at the back of this book for our recommendations.

Maintain a List of Reliable Websites

Cyberspace provides quite a few diabetes websites. Be wary of the medical information they offer. Most sites are focused on promoting various products and may not be monitored by medical professionals for safety or accuracy. Take care when participating in chat rooms or unmonitored bulletin boards. Unfortunately, some folks enjoy posting misinformation; false diabetes treatments, dangerous cures, and misleading information abound.

Remember the Aspartame and canola oil rumors? In December, 1998, a bizarre note was posted on the Internet that accused the sweetener Aspartame (also known as Nutra-

Sweet® and Equal®) of being extremely toxic to humans. All these comments were absolutely untrue, but, unfortunately, this rumor still persists. It is true that some individuals cannot tolerate Aspartame, but fatal disease has never been linked with its use.

The canola oil rumor viciously and incorrectly accuses this healthy oil of being a poisonous substance causing emphysema, anemia, constipation, irritability, and blindness. Again, totally false. Why do people post these lies? Just like graffiti writers who deface buildings, they do it because they can.

Be part of the solution. Don't believe or spread ridiculous rumors. If you read something that sounds suspicious or too good to be true, check its accuracy by visiting www.urbanlegends.about.com; www.quackwatch.com; or any website that debunks false Internet claims. Check with your healthcare provider before trying out any advice you have read.

See Suggested Resources at the back of this book for a list of recommended websites, magazines, books, and other educational materials.

Attend a Diabetes Education Program

Go often to keep up with changes. A session at your local hospital will give you an opportunity to check the value of diabetes information you have heard about and want to try. Invite your family to join you.

Programming varies, but most hospitals have group classes to review the basics of diabetes, meal planning, and other lifestyle topics. As an example, Baptist Hospital of South Florida currently offers these classes:

- CADRE (Cardiovascular and Diabetes Risk Eradication). A weight-loss and exercise program specifically designed for people who are at high risk for developing either cardiovascular disease or diabetes.

- Dia-Beat-It. A personalized weight-control program designed especially for adults with diabetes, pre-diabetes, or insulin-resistance syndrome.

- Parent/Child Diabetes Support Group. A session for children who have diabetes and their parents.

Many hospitals also offer insulin-pump support groups and classes. Group sessions offer you an opportunity to meet others in your community who are also learning to live with diabetes. You have a chance to ask questions, clarify misinformation, and get answers.

Review All Information with Your Healthcare Team

Don't alter your diabetes treatment because of something you read online or heard from a neighbor. Rumors run rampant and should be checked out with your healthcare team before being accepted as fact. Neighbors may mean well, but new developments have dramatically changed treatment and care in recent years. It is not your "grandfather's diabetes" any longer. Complications are not as common as they once were, meal planning is much more relaxed, and medication treatments allow for lots of lifestyle flexibility.

Before you share information with your healthcare providers, ask yourself these questions:

1. *Is this information from a reputable source?*

Examine the background of the authors. Are they affiliated with a recognized medical organization or diabetes center? Several quality organizations include:

- American Diabetes Association (ADA)

- American Heart Association (AHA)

- Diabetes Research Institute (DRI)

- Joslin Diabetes Center

- Juvenile Diabetes Research Foundation International (JDRF)

- TCOYD (Taking Control of Your Diabetes)

- A major university

2. *Do the authors have respected credentials?*

Most writers of medical articles have a generous "alphabet soup" of initials following their names. These abbreviations stand for various educational or professional achievements that indicate certain levels of expertise. If you are puzzled by someone's credentials, request additional information.

Profession	Initials	Definitions
Diabetes Specialists	CDE	Certified Diabetes Educator
	BC-ADM	Board Certified-Advanced Diabetes Manager
Physicians	MD	Medical Doctor
	DO	Doctor of Osteopathic Medicine
Registered Dietitians	RD	Registered Dietitian
	LD/N or LD	Passed exam in state that requires licensure
Podiatrists	DPM	Doctor of Podiatric Medicine
Nurses	RN	Registered Nurse
Mental Health Professionals	PhD	Doctor of Philosophy (Psychology)
	MSW	Master of Social Work (Social Worker)
	LCSW	Licensed Clinical Social Worker
Pharmacists	RPH	Registered Parmacist
	PharmD	Doctor of Pharmacy

Definitely watch for the certification CDE, which indicates a Certified Diabetes Educator. Healthcare professionals, including doctors, nurses, dietitians, podiatrists, pharmacists, exercise specialists, psychiatrists, social workers, therapists and others, must complete a rigorous and comprehensive exam before they are eligible to use the CDE initials. This highly respected certification is difficult to attain and indicates an expertise in diabetes care and education. If the author of a publication is a CDE, you are probably in very capable hands.

3. *Is the magazine or journal respected?*

Most quality publications list members of their advisory boards at the beginning of each issue. Review their names, affiliations, and credentials.

4. *Is the website reputable?*

Don't be swayed by "website awards." Awards are usually given for website design and do not guarantee that all of the posted information is reliable and safe. See if the website has a qualified diabetes educator on staff or is associated with a recognized and respected health organization.

We would like to believe that all healthcare providers welcome their patients' participation in decisions that affect their treatment. But what if your doctor is not open to new ideas or interested in what you bring into the office to discuss? In that case, here are some alternatives:

1. Respect the fact that you may have a difference of opinion about a supplement or treatment choice. Listen to what your healthcare provider has to say.

2. Bring quality articles that provide information on the topics you wish to discuss.

3. If you can't discuss it openly and honestly, seek another opinion.

4. Are you being seen by a doctor who specializes in diabetes? If your diabetes is being treated by a family physician or internist, he or she may not have the time to stay current with the rapidly changing treatment options that occur almost daily. A diabetes specialist can be either an endocrinologist or a diabetologist. You deserve the best and most up to date care possible. Make every effort to see an appropriate specialist.

WHAT A PERSON WITH DIABETES MAY WANT HIS OR HER FRIENDS TO KNOW

1. I don't want people to judge me based on diabetes information they have heard from others; these assumptions are often wrong.

2. Diabetes is a serious disease. I hope others will respect my needs and not urge me to eat unhealthy foods.

3. Hey, I'm not ready to be buried yet. With good care, I can have a long and healthy life.

4. I don't want to be hassled about my diabetes. This condition can be frustrating and confusing for all of us, friends and loved ones alike. If you want to help, ask me directly what you can do. I welcome your help.

5. I want to be treated like anyone else; just because I have diabetes doesn't mean I've become fragile or stupid.

WHAT A LOVED ONE MAY WANT THE PERSON WITH DIABETES TO KNOW

1. I may not fully understand diabetes, but I'm trying to. I hope that I won't make ignorant comments, but if I do, please understand and be willing to explain.

2. I want to learn more about diabetes. Let me know if I can join you at your appointments and classes.

3. I don't mean to nag you. I care about you and am worried about your health.

You and those you love may have very different beliefs about diabetes. Some of these differences can affect your relationships. Do your relatives blame you for developing diabetes? Do friends urge you to stick to unproven dietary regimens? Perhaps you are following questionable diabetes practices. Once you separate truth from fiction, you and your loved ones can find meaningful ways to support each other when diabetes enters your relationship.

Chapter 2

Even Robin Needed His Merry Men

Diabetes is much easier to handle when you have friends and family rooting for you. A loving spouse, loyal friend, or true-blue coworker can offer so much. They are your exercise partners, they cheer for you when you meet challenging diabetes goals, and they listen to you gripe after a lousy day. They also accompany you to diabetes classes and doctors' appointments. Most of all, these terrific folks remind you that you're an important human being with a tremendous amount to share, not just a person with a disease. Their emotional backing helps you succeed where others, who lack support, may fail.

The Two Types of Support

Emotional support is listening and hugging. It's a shoulder to cry on and a kind smile. Your supporters provide a "high-five" when you meet an elusive weight or blood glucose goal. They help you make it through a rough day.

> I don't know where I would be without my big sister, Letty. She worries about me and my diabetes when I don't worry about myself. I was diagnosed with type 1 two years ago as a senior in college, and she has been there since day one. I count on her to help me when I'm about to give up. We discuss our frustrations during long phone conversations and she helps me put things back into perspective.
>
> —Katie

Hands-on support is tangible. It includes actions that help you implement your diabetes care plan. Hands-on supporters may:

a. Accompany you to a doctor's appointment.

b. Prepare and share diabetes-friendly foods with you.

c. Pick up your prescriptions.

d. Assist with daily foot inspections.

e. Watch your kids while you attend a diabetes program.

DOROTHY AND BILL

Dorothy is terrified of needles. Her doctor said that she needs to take insulin injections to control her type 2 diabetes. Fortunately, her husband Bill has offered to give her all of her shots. This isn't the most practical solution, but until Dorothy builds up her confidence level and begins doing her own injections, Bill's helping hand will be exactly what she needs to bring her blood sugar levels under control.

JARED AND TOBY

Jared woke up feeling lousy and quickly became worried that he might be low. His wife Toby sat down at the foot of the bed and waited patiently as Jared completed his morning glucose check. "Darn, I knew it! I'm low again. I just hate this. I'm so mad at myself. I have to stop doing this." Without a word, Toby reached over to the nightstand and handed Jared a juice box to drink to treat his hypoglycemia (low blood sugar). He could handle it himself, but having her nearby made him feel so much better. The juice did the trick, and both Jared and Toby felt better about starting the day.

When loved ones root for you, it improves your ability to handle the daunting challenges of diabetes self-care. You are not weak if someone helps you. Dorothy is lucky to have

Bill, who rolls up his sleeves and helps her take action. Someone in your life can help you manage your diabetes more easily, too.

How to Enlist Support

"If you don't ask, you don't get." Unfortunately, asking does not always guarantee that support will come. Are you looking to others for assistance but not receiving the help that you want? Perhaps you should ask in a different way.

Be specific. Don't use general phrases like, "I need your help." Friends are not mind readers. They can't anticipate your every need. Ask them to help with things such as clearing unhealthy foods from your cupboards. Be as specific as possible.

Check your emotions at the door. Make requests as dispassionately as possible. When you ask for help, don't sound angry or accusing. Don't nag family members because they forgot to pick up your prescriptions or forgot to call to ask about your recent doctor's appointment. People are less likely to help if you yell at them or put them down. How would you respond if someone asked you in that way? Set a time to discuss your feelings, if desired, but don't color your requests with unresolved anger.

Who can you ask for help with your diabetes care? Here's a partial list:

- Spouse
- Friends
- Children
- Relatives
- Coworkers
- Workout partners
- Neighbors

Tell potential supporters about your diabetes and see how they react. If they are responsive, follow your explanation with a concrete and clear request. Would you like help with food preparation? Do you need someone to shop for items on your meal plan? How about a cheerleader to help you stick to your workout schedule? Think about the type of assistance you need. You can manage your diabetes without supportive family and friends, but they certainly can make life easier!

If you don't have a doting spouse handy or a direct line to a sister, what are your options? How can you get the support you desire to help you handle the challenges of living with diabetes?

Local Support Groups

What comes to mind when you think of a support group? You may recall "The Bob Newhart Show," in which Newhart played a therapist who ran a group filled with wacky characters. One sat knitting, one complained non-stop, and another had such an ego that the rest of the group couldn't stand him. Your local diabetes support group may have some colorful characters, but it will be nothing like the show. Different people come together to share their diabetes concerns and successes, not to drive each other crazy.

Diabetes support groups are often held monthly at local hospitals or community centers and are usually free or a small donation is requested. You have no obligation to come each time. Groups offer many benefits:

- They can help you feel less isolated
- They can make you more comfortable and confident with your diabetes
- You'll hear about different treatment options

- You'll learn how others handle family, work, and other social challenges

- You will meet others like you

What a difference it makes to exchange thoughts and ideas with those who have "been there, done that." Certain conditions, however, will not be resolved by simply sharing them with others. Issues such as depression or severe anxiety require sessions with a skilled professional.

It's easy to locate support groups in your area:

- Ask a member of your healthcare team

- Call a local hospital. Support groups often meet there

- Contact a nearby university

- Contact your city's community center

- E-mail the American Diabetes Association at www.diabetes.org or call 1-800-DIABETES

- Call any diabetes organization in your area such as the Juvenile Diabetes Research Foundation

- Search on the Internet

- Watch for diabetes fundraising projects and walk-a-thons. Participants may know about programs in your neighborhood

- Ask a friend who also has diabetes. Perhaps you can go together

Not all groups will meet your needs. If necessary, try several groups until you find a comfortable mix of people. One may have too few participants in your age group, or you may prefer a group with more insulin pump users. Fortunately, many different types of diabetes support groups exist.

An Internet search for "Diabetes Support Groups Tulsa Oklahoma" brought up 24 locations, including Jane Phillips Medical Center, Claremore Indian Hospital, and the Diabetes Center of Oklahoma at INTEGRIS Baptist Medical Center. Not a bad start. If you live in a more remote area, locate groups in your locality by using the contact options listed above. If you don't find a group in your area, start one. You'll help so many people, including yourself.

Diabetes Classes, Conferences, and Seminars

A local diabetes class is another great place for developing supportive friendships. The skills of the teacher are most important. Many are adept at motivating attendees to participate in discussions. They know how to make the sessions both educational and fun. If your session runs the entire day, or over a period of several days, shared meals and activities will bond your group together. Hospital-based programs generally charge a fee, but your insurance may pay for part or all of it.

Numerous diabetes conferences and seminars are available throughout the year. For example, Taking Control of Your Diabetes (www.tcoyd.org) is a not-for-profit organization that puts on motivational conferences and health fairs around the country each year. The ADA plans health fair expos as well (www.diabetes.org). Attend as many as possible. They will keep you motivated and up to date on the most recent advances.

Subscribe to Diabetes Magazines

Diabetes magazines such as *Diabetes Forecast*, the official publication of the American Diabetes Association, offer community connections and provide pen pal information. *Diabetes Forecast*'s "Making Friends" section is located at the back of each issue and features three categories: Friends 18–29, Friends 30–49, and Friends 50 and Over. To find a pen pal, write to Making Friends, ADA, 1701 N. Beauregard Street, Alexandria, VA 22311.

Other excellent magazines are:

Diabetes Health (formerly *Diabetes Interview*)

Diabetes Positive!

Diabetes Self-Management

Internet Chat Groups and Bulletin Boards

A chat room contains live online "discussion" that offers real communal interaction. Registered participants type in their thoughts, which post almost immediately on-screen. You can join in or just read along. Because chats are live, inappropriate information can be posted quickly and easily, so beware of dangerous or incorrect advice. Some chat rooms invite experts to appear at scheduled times to interact with online participants; many are very worthwhile.

Visit www.childrenwithdiabetes.com, a website for children and adults with diabetes, as well as their friends and families. It routinely hosts expert chat sessions. Past chats have featured Nicole Johnson, Miss America 1999, and Mr. Food, who discussed holiday food items.

Insulin pump users can try www.insulin-pumpers.org, which usually hosts chat sessions in the evening.

Internet bulletin boards provide static conversation. Just like the old cork board that hangs in your kitchen, you post a message and wait for a response. Comments may appear immediately, or they might be posted several weeks or even months later. The following are just a few of the sites that have bulletin boards:

- diabetes.org—website of the American Diabetes Association

- diabetic.com—a sales site whose bulletin board is monitored by a CDE (Certified Diabetes Educator)

- jdrf.org—the Juvenile Diabetes Research Foundation

- joslin.org—the Joslin Diabetes Center

Check with your healthcare team before trying any advice that you find on the Internet.

Identify—and Get—the Support You Need

Do you know what kind of support you need? That can actually be very difficult to determine. Here are some individuals who discovered their need and found a way to support it:

Identify the issue

Dan and Debbie enjoyed exercising together, but when her work schedule changed and her trips out of town became more frequent, Dan felt lost. He didn't like to bike or walk alone and quickly lost interest in both activities. His diabetes control began to suffer and his weight began to climb. At first, he blamed himself for his terrible lack of willpower, but then he realized it was much easier to be active when he could share it with someone. With Debbie's help, he decided it was time to get creative.

Now find the support

Dan called a few friends and set up a weekly racquetball game and bike ride through the neighborhood. He also signed up for a yoga class at a nearby gym. Regular exercise helped him control his blood sugar levels and improve his overall health. He also developed a new support system of workout buddies.

Those who assist you don't have to live nearby. Don't underestimate the power of a long-distance phone conversation.

Suzanne was in a slump. She has had type 2 diabetes for about four months and was starting to lose her desire to wake up and complete her workout before leaving for work. She phoned her sister, Lisa. They don't live in the same city, but they push each other to stick to their respective exercise schedules. Most conversations are filled with family gossip, but today Suzanne really needed Lisa's help. Fortunately, the call did the trick. Lisa charged her sister up by challenging her to set a new goal. Suzanne loved the idea, put on her walking shoes, and headed out the door.

Identify the issue

Ned can't check his feet each day. He is not as flexible as he used to be and is unable to bring his leg up high enough to inspect it properly and spot new cuts or infections. He has tried using a mirror, but prefers to have someone help him.

Now find the support

Ned's teenage granddaughter Leslie visits his apartment several times a week. He never thought to ask her to do his foot checks. "I can't bother her; she has a life of her own. I'm grateful that she visits at all." Ned finally asked, and Leslie was happy to help. He showed her the proper way to inspect his feet and even provided her with a small plastic filament to check his sensitivity. "I sure appreciate the help!" he told her.

Now you give it a try:

Identify the issue

Jot down a diabetes-related activity that you would like some help doing. Be as specific as possible.

Now find the support

Like Ned, think of someone, or several people, who can help you do this activity. When ready, contact them and get the support you deserve.

"Supportive" Sabotage

Unfortunately, not all support is helpful.

> My family is angry at me about my diabetes. I weigh almost 300 pounds and was diagnosed with type 2 about three months ago. I have a husband and three boys ages 15, 17, and 21. I don't always feel well, so they throw their own brand of advice at me: "Come on. Stop whining and just deal with it." They really think this is helpful. My husband thinks that such comments will "snap me out of it." This isn't the help that I want. I just don't know what to do.
>
> —Dora

Dora's family means well, but their "support" isn't supportive at all. In fact, it makes Dora feel even more discouraged. It is easy to understand their frustration and anger, but blaming Dora for her diabetes just makes things worse. Unfortunately, they don't really know how to help.

Some saboteurs, like Dora's family, verbalize their attitudes. Some say nothing at all.

TERRY AND RON

> My wife, Terry, takes care of her diabetes all by herself. She has been doing that since I've known her, about 12 years. She got diabetes when she was very little. She has the type that needs the shots. I don't ask about it and don't deal with it. Actually, I don't even want to hear about it. The needles, the complications that go with it, I just prefer that she not tell me about it.

And then there are those who offer negative support with a smile:

KITTY

Kitty sat quietly on the couch sipping a diet Coke at the family reunion. "Come on, Kit, a little cake won't hurt," said her cousin David. *But it will,* she thought. Soon the whole family was standing around urging her to take a taste of Aunt Joan's six-layer chocolate-coconut masterpiece. "She put a lot of work into it," added her husband, Stewart.

Kitty felt terribly embarrassed and decided that a little taste wouldn't hurt. But that "little taste" made her seethe with anger inside. She had promised herself that she would stick to her meal plan and get serious about her weight loss goals. With that small bite melting in her mouth, she decided to suspend her diet for the day. She went directly into the kitchen and took an even larger second piece.

BEN AND JOAN

The phone rang in Ben's office. "Ben-Ben, I just left work. Skip your exercise today and go see a movie with me." Ben and Joan had just started dating. She knew that he had diabetes, but she didn't fully understand what it meant. He didn't want to take this lovely invitation and turn it into a lecture on diabetes, exercise, and his personal care schedule. "OK," answered Ben. "Meet you downstairs in 15 minutes."

Such well-meaning and loving comments disrespect the diabetes needs of each of these individuals. Negative support, even if unintentional, can cause the following damage:

a. Reduce your confidence

b. Harm your self-esteem

c. Push you to neglect important diabetes tasks

d. Make you too uncomfortable to care for your diabetes when others are around

e. Cause you to ignore important symptoms because you don't want to be a complainer

f. Cause you to delay seeking assistance for an urgent situation because you don't want to bother anyone

g. Cause you to resent your diabetes and your loved ones

How can you overcome these awkward situations?

Kitty and Ben have to find a way to better communicate their needs. Here are some suggestions:

Options for Kitty:

1. Eat prior to the next family party. It is easier to say no to a dessert when you aren't very hungry.

2. Give yourself permission to have a small sliver of cake. Follow it with a tall glass of diet soda and enjoy the evening.

3. Bring your own special dessert to the next event and share it with others.

4. Practice phrases that clearly convey your message. For example: "The cake looks amazing, but I'll have to pass. Thanks anyway." Or "Just a small slice, please."

Options for Ben:

1. Invite Joan to share a workout instead of a movie.

2. Review your workout schedule with Joan. Plan future activities around it.

3. Practice your message and use it when needed. For example: "I'd love to skip exercise and go to a film with you, but my body won't let me. Can we go to a later show?"

If encounters with your family become too disruptive, consider meeting with a mental health professional to discuss the situation and find additional solutions. Most of all, don't give up. Your health is important and others will go along with you if you are strong and confident.

WHAT A PERSON WITH DIABETES MAY WANT HIS OR HER FRIENDS TO KNOW

1. It isn't always easy to live with diabetes. I want to have supportive friends and family around who understand and appreciate my concerns but also don't make too big a deal out of all of this.

2. I may ask you for assistance, but only if I need it.

3. I may prefer to do some of my diabetes tasks alone. Please don't take any offense if I don't ask you for help or accept help from someone else.

WHAT A LOVED ONE MAY WANT THE PERSON WITH DIABETES TO KNOW

1. I want to help you sometimes, but I also have errands to run and things that I must do. I will try to be available, but I can't always be there for you.

2. If you ask too much of me, I will get overwhelmed. Find other individuals to help also.

3. I feel important and needed when there are ways I can support your efforts, so please let me.

4. I can't read your mind and may not realize that you need assistance. Ask me for help if you need it.

5. I like being of help, especially when you appreciate my efforts. A "thank you" makes me feel very special.

Yes, even Robin Hood had his merry men—Little John, Friar Tuck, and the rest—who worked together to achieve their common goal: Rob from the rich to give to the poor. Robin might have been able to achieve this alone, but having the assistance of his merry men made his task much easier. Research shows that positive and encouraging support makes a difference in your diabetes care.

Find ways to bring others into your circle of support. Imagine yourself in the middle, independent and strong, while the circle around you is filled with those who want to help you stay that way. Don't deny yourself this rich source of support, and don't deny your loved ones the opportunity to help you. Inviting them to join you in your healthier lifestyle is a gift that you all can share.

Chapter 3

Diabetes Police and Diabetes Criminals

Do friends and relatives nag you about your diabetes care? Do they act like members of a secret police force and monitor every morsel you eat and every blood test you take? If you love someone with diabetes, do you offer suggestions or get upset even when you know it will make things worse? Unsolicited advice is tough to handle, especially when it involves something as personal as diabetes. On the other hand, it is tough to stay quiet when someone you care about seems to ignore his or her medical needs.

Noted "Galloping Gourmet" Graham Kerr has been married to his wife Treena since 1955. The following is a personal "police moment" from their new book, *Charting a Course to Wellness* (ADA, 2004), which details their life story, how they handled Treena's heart attack, high blood pressure, and diabetes, plus a generous number of wonderful recipes.

> One day in 1978, I had been reading about the nitrite and saturated fat content in bologna sausage and went straight from this alarming (and well overstated) report to see my beloved Treena putting . . . yes . . . bologna into our son Andy's sandwich.
>
> "You're not putting that in our son's sandwich." I was pointing my finger at the sausage as it hung limply in her hand.
>
> Suddenly Treena snapped. She is, after all, a direct descendant of the Queen of the Romanian Gypsies. She flung the bologna in my direction. It makes quite a good Frisbee. It fell at my feet. She then did something quite hard to

replicate (the object of good science?). She dealt the rest of the sticky pack like a Vegas card dealer . . . all over the floor.

She turned to the pantry cupboard, picking up random packets and jars and throwing them into the trashcan whilst shouting, "There's nothing in the world left to eat with you!"

We lived between Liberace and Kirk Douglas and Treena has great voice projection. This obviously concerned me greatly since I still felt my reputation as a "gourmet" was in immediate danger.

Now I believe that men are really quite sensitive and have considerable discernment at times like this and I definitely had the feeling that something was wrong.

"Tell you what," I cried out above all the din.

"What," Treena blazed back.

"I'll cook what you like to eat and eat what I like. We'll have two styles," I placated.

"Fine, fine," she replied.

You always know when you've got a deal with Treena.

Why do they do it? What compels husbands, wives, parents, siblings, children, friends, acquaintances, neighbors, coworkers, medical professionals, and even total strangers to brazenly offer unwanted advice? Most want to help but don't know how to do it constructively. They feel that if they don't comment and point out your diabetes shortcomings, they will be accomplices in your downfall.

What Is Your Role?

Do you recognize yourself in this drama? Are you a diabetes police officer? Do you offer unsolicited, aggravating comments to the ones you love? Or are you the target, the one being treated like a criminal? Read below and see.

If you are a card-carrying member of the Diabetes Police, you might say:

1. "If you'd just stop eating so much, your diabetes would get better."

2. "Your blood sugar is high again. What did you do wrong *this* time?"

3. "You seem upset; check your blood sugar."

4. "The doctor told you to exercise. Won't you at least try?"

5. "My wife (husband, son, daughter, friend) can't eat that. She has diabetes."

6. "Why won't you do what the doctor says? Don't you care about your health?"

Or are you a Diabetes Criminal?

1. Do you snack in private to make sure that no one bugs you?

2. When you check your blood sugar, do you often hide the results if your numbers are high?

3. Do you feel angry whenever anyone makes negative comments about your diabetes?

4. Do you sometimes do the opposite of what a loved one suggests, such as eating more if you are told to eat less?

5. When someone asks about your health, do you say "I'm fine" even when you're not?

6. Do others often criticize your diabetes control?

7. Do others treat you as if you were fragile or stupid just because you have diabetes?

8. Be honest—do you ever neglect your diabetes care?

The diabetes police infiltrated the happy home of Jeff and Nancy. They have been married for three years, and Jeff's diabetes has brought a lot of tension into their relationship. Nancy says:

I can't help it, I try to stay out of Jeff's diabetes, but what can I do when he won't exercise? He promises to lose weight but raids the kitchen after I go to bed. I try to hold my tongue, I really do. I even pinch my arm to remind myself to keep quiet. But that little voice in my head screams out and says, "You are Jeff's wife. If you don't say anything, who will?" I'm angry an awful lot about this and blurt out comments that I shouldn't say. I want our relationship to be about us, not Jeff's diabetes.

Nancy is in a tough spot. Her desire to help her husband stay healthy is heartfelt, but her frustration has turned into anger. Nancy desires a healthy marriage and a healthy husband. She wants to be Jeff's loving and supportive wife, not his nagging mother.

Jeff responds:

Nancy doesn't understand. I am caring for my diabetes as best I can. She gets upset with whatever I do. I hate her nagging and don't like to be told what to do. I sometimes do unhealthy things just because she tells me not to. Nancy needs to let me care for my diabetes in my own way and accept me as I am.

Diabetes isn't easy. It affects every moment with no days off. Some people control it better than others, but all must stay vigilant. If Nancy and Jeff's behavior toward each other continues, it could destroy their relationship.

Negative police/criminal behaviors can:

1. Discourage open and honest communication

2. Cause frustration for both parties

3. Reduce the desire for intimacy

4. Cause a person to ignore important diabetes needs

5. Encourage a partner to withdraw from the relationship

6. Drive a person to seek support elsewhere

7. Sever the relationship altogether

Do you have a "police officer" in your life? How can you stop him or her from hovering over your every move? If you are a member of the police force, how can you keep your heartfelt concern from destroying your relationship?

Here are three activities that might help: the Behavior Bargain, the Informal Bargain, and "Beam Me Up, Scotty!"

The Behavior Bargain

Rules: For exactly one week, begin and continue a positive behavior if your partner promises to stop a negative one.

Goal: Have fun while achieving positive behavior change.

Nagging is very one-sided. One of you plays the all-knowing partner while the other receives the criticism. The Behavior Bargain levels the playing field. In this activity, both partners agree to maintain their behavior changes for one week. To start, create a list of possible behavior changes.

Step 1: Identify Police/Criminal Behaviors

Jeff and Nancy begin their Behavior Bargain with a romantic candlelight dinner. This is a time for sharing, not accusing. No negative comments allowed. The goal is to remove tension from your relationship. During the evening, they list the behaviors that each finds troubling.

Jeff's List— I don't appreciate it when Nancy:

1. Searches my pockets and car for candy wrappers

2. Reminds me to exercise

3. Shares my diabetes problems with my family

4. Fills my desk with diabetes articles

5. Tells the waiter to seat us quickly because I have diabetes and need to eat

Nancy's List— I don't appreciate it when Jeff:

1. Buys unhealthy foods away from home

2. Doesn't follow the doctor's orders

3. Becomes angry when I ask his family to help with his diabetes care

Now create your own list. You can use some of the complaints stated above, but try to come up with grievances that are personal and unique to your own situation.

Step 2: The Bargain Begins

Choose a positive behavior to implement when your partner stops a negative one. Here is what Jeff and Nancy did.

Jeff begins his part of the bargain with a positive behavior. He promises to use the treadmill for 15 minutes on Monday, Wednesday, and Friday evenings while watching Larry King on CNN. That is his positive choice.

Nancy promises to end a negative behavior. She offers to stop discussing Jeff's diabetes with other members of the family. They agree to keep this bargain for exactly one week. Do the same with the behaviors you choose.

Step 3: The Results

The week is over and it's time to celebrate—Jeff and Nancy met their goals. Jeff fit his exercise easily into his schedule and actually enjoys doing it. His blood sugar improved and he now sleeps better at night. Nancy didn't realize how many diabetes details she was sharing with her relatives. Staying mum on the topic makes her feel less like the town gossip and more like a loving wife who respects her husband's privacy. Both are proud of their accomplishment. They decide to continue this bargain for another week and take on another bargain when ready. You can do the same.

Rewarding Success

Behavior change is difficult and deserves a celebration. The following is a list of rewards that Jeff and Nancy plan for themselves each time they complete a successful week of behavior bargains.

Rent a video

Go out to a movie

Attend a concert

Take a romantic stroll

Give each other foot massages

Play chess, cards, or a favorite board game

Go for a bike ride

The Informal Bargain

The Behavior Bargain can also be done in a less formal way with friends, relatives, and acquaintances.

Rules: Offer to begin a positive behavior if your friend or relative stops a negative one.

Goal: Achieve positive behavior change and reduce tensions.

This approach skips the formal list-making session. You offer to make a change and hope that your friend will respond. Here are some possible scenarios.

A parent criticizes your behavior:

"Mom, let's try this—if you stop mentioning my weight, I will cut out my after-dinner snacking. Agreed? Let's try it."

Your brother treats you like the village idiot:

Each week, when you and your brother play softball, he repeatedly asks how you are feeling and cautions all on the field to be careful since you have diabetes and wear an insulin pump. You suggest the following:

"Roger, my pump is totally safe and so am I. Let's make a deal. If you stop making these comments, I promise to let you know if I need any assistance."

You wish to help out a friend who has diabetes:

"Tom, I know my comments bug you, but I do care. How can I help you with all of the diabetes duties you have to do? Let's make a deal. If I stop commenting on the foods you choose, you and I could walk every morning before work. Heck, it would be good for me as well as for you."

Beam Me Up, Scotty! (or Get Me Out of Here!)

Rules: Anticipate negative comments or behaviors, and award yourself points when you guess behaviors correctly.

Goal: Achieve emotional distance from the situation.

Wouldn't life be simple if you could ask Star Trek's Chief Engineer, Scotty, to beam you back to your spaceship whenever someone criticized you? Since that can't happen, this exercise does the next best thing. It removes you, mentally, from the role of victim and transports you into the role of spectator.

1. *Anticipate the comments or behaviors.*

Before a challenging encounter, anticipate what that difficult person will say to you. For example, your coworker Roger always comments on how tired you look and asks if your blood sugar is low. (His brother has diabetes, so he claims to know all about it.) Or whenever you visit, Aunt Betty always brings out a tray of thickly frosted cookies. You've tried speaking to her, but nothing will change her ways, regardless of what you say or do.

2. *Keep score (or just enjoy the game).*

Now enter the room and wait. If Roger comments on your fatigued look and diabetes control, award yourself a point. Good job, you guessed well! If Aunt Betty brings out her famous desserts right on cue, award yourself another point. Not bad, you're on a roll. If they don't make the anticipated remark, no points are awarded. Before you know it, you'll be laughing inside as a spectator and no longer taking their words to heart. You really don't have to keep score; your attitude shift will be reward enough. They will still comment, but your anxiety level will be lower, which will make the situation less frustrating. Thank them and laugh it off. Remember, you can't change anyone's behavior but your own. Do the best you can, and if they don't like it, *it is their problem*!

I use this technique a lot. I have had type 2 diabetes for about three years. I've been married for about 12 years and

my relationship with my mother-in-law has never been something to brag about. Now I have diabetes and she has even
more to comment on. She criticizes my diabetes care whenever I visit—I drink too much juice, I look too heavy, etc. I
always leave hurt and upset. While driving over to her home,
I now anticipate the comments that she might make. I even
share my thoughts with my husband. You should see the
looks on our faces when the expected comments come out.
What an improvement! I feel so much better.

—Laurie

Here is Diane's story.

I always went crazy when Keith arrived home and caught
me on the couch eating chips and watching television instead
of working out. He would make a nasty comment and start a
horrible fight. I have had type 2 diabetes for two years and
want to take care of myself, but I have to do it at my own
pace, not Keith's.

I love Keith but hate his nagging. I tried the "Beam Me
Up, Scotty" activity. It made such a difference. First, I anticipated what Keith would say when he got home. If he made a
crack about me and the couch, I didn't argue back—he was
doing exactly what I expected. Because I stopped arguing, he
stopped making comments. Without that pressure, I am exercising more, and we both see the results.

It is best to work out your problems, but a temporary
escape, like the above activity suggests, can sometimes be helpful, especially when you know the situation cannot change. Diabetes is challenging enough without the intrusion of the Diabetes Police. Here is a checklist of things that can help both you
and the ones you love become a more supportive team.

Your Anti-Diabetes-Police Checklist

—Get the Facts

Most experts define good diabetes control as having
an A1C value of less than 7 percent and blood pressure below 130/80. (The A1C test measures your average blood

sugar levels for the past two to three months.) If your healthcare team agrees that your control is good, that speaks volumes. Share your good results with your police force and let them know you are doing just fine.

— Be Honest

Speak with your diabetes police officers about your frustrations. Let them know that you appreciate their concern but their behavior isn't helpful, makes you feel uncomfortable, and won't help you manage your diabetes. Be assertive. Don't blame them, but do let them know that you are in charge of your diabetes care, and no one else.

—Go Public

Let the police see that you do care for your diabetes. Invite a loved one to watch you check your blood sugar level and then say how you plan to treat it. Or discuss the various tasks that you do each day to keep your diabetes controlled. When you share this kind of information, you reassure your nagging police force that you know what you are doing and are acting responsibly.

—Redirect Their Efforts

Thank everyone for their concern, and suggest constructive ways that they can help you. For example, if your wife accuses you of eating too much "junk," ask her to help you fill the cupboard with healthier choices.

—Review Your Own Behavior

Do you care for your diabetes in the best way possible? Perhaps your family is right about your lack of attention to your health and tried to tell you gently but must now yell to get your attention. Think about what they are saying. Maybe it is time for you to take better control of your diabetes and make a few changes.

—Seek Professional Help

If you have tried everything to end the tension between you and your police officers but nothing has worked,
suggest a meeting of those involved with a mental health
professional to help end the battle. Your healthcare provider
should be able to recommend a qualified individual.

—Will More Education Help?

To be fair, your diabetes police won't necessarily stop
bugging you just because they become well-informed about
diabetes. In some cases, it could make things even worse! But
when you and your loved ones both learn the real facts about
diabetes, when you are all privy to what is needed—and not
needed—then you have laid the important groundwork for
understanding, meaningful conversation, and the possibility
of true teamwork.

WHAT A PERSON WITH DIABETES MAY WANT HIS OR HER FRIENDS TO KNOW

1. I hate people treating me like I'm fragile. I don't
   need to have the hostess at the restaurant think that
   we must be seated quickly because I have diabetes. I
   don't want to skip the dessert menu because others
   think that it is too tempting for me. It isn't.

2. I need support, not unsolicited advice. Diabetes can
   be challenging and I'd like to know that everyone is
   there for me, but I do know what I am supposed to
   do. I will ask for help if I need it.

3. I don't respond well to lectures. This is my life and I
   am doing the best I can do right now. I know that
   you all mean well, but please skip the lectures. I don't
   want to hear stories about your aunt who lost her leg
   to diabetes and your neighbor's niece who was recently diagnosed.

WHAT A LOVED ONE MAY WANT THE PERSON WITH DIABETES TO KNOW

1. When I bug you, I do it out of love.

2. I get scared when I see you are having difficulties with your diabetes.

3. I know you think it is none of my business, but I'd like to be reassured from time to time that you are taking good care of your diabetes.

4. Let me know what you need so I won't have to bother you by asking.

Don't allow a brutal police/criminal tug-of-war ruin the relationship that you and your loved ones share. Try the activities listed above and visit a mental health professional who understands diabetes if your difficulties become greater than you can handle on your own. Don't give up. Find what works for you.

Chapter 4

Like a Pebble in a Pond

Drop a pebble into a small pool of water and watch what happens. Within moments, ripples spread throughout the entire area. The disturbing feelings that often accompany diabetes do the very same thing. They affect you and eventually touch those around you. If you find diabetes difficult to handle, take a good look at your underlying feelings. How do you view your diabetes? Once you understand the real facts and learn how to make peace with the disease, you and everyone close to you will find it so much easier to live with diabetes.

> When I was first diagnosed with type 2 diabetes, I cried for three nights straight. I even posted a message on a diabetes internet bulletin board pleading for help. Why did I have to get it? How was I going to support my wife, mother, and three lovely daughters? If I died, how would my family survive? I feel more confident now that I know more about diabetes, but those early days were really tough.
>
> —Carlos

It is normal to have strong emotions such as fear, depression, anger, frustration, and guilt when diabetes enters your world. Some come from the worries and aggravations of living with a chronic illness. Others may have more to do with your physical condition—such as the irritability, fatigue, anger, and other feelings that can develop when large blood sugar swings overwhelm your body.

Of course, it is possible to have diabetes and not feel particularly bothered by it. Many individuals who enjoy problem-solving rise to the challenges that diabetes offers each day. However you feel about it, having diabetes is not your fault.

> Lots of overweight folks eat whatever they want but don't get diabetes. My entire family is also overweight, yet none of them have it. I'm the only one who got type 2 diabetes. What did I do wrong?
>
> —Sandra

You may have strong or even painful feelings about diabetes—that is understandable. If your feelings aren't too overwhelming, they can sometimes be helpful, especially if they inspire you to take positive action. Being frightened about long-term complications, for example, may lead you to take a more active role in your diabetes care. Becoming aggravated because your best efforts don't seem to have improved your glucose control could motivate you to enroll in a diabetes education program and learn techniques that will make a difference.

Ignoring feelings can cause them to intensify and, over a long period of time, create even bigger problems:

a. You might become more irritable, restless or impatient.

b. You might find it harder to concentrate at certain times.

c. You may lose your appetite.

d. You may become increasingly tired and lethargic.

e. You could start to have difficulty sleeping.

f. Your body may hurt—muscle aches, headaches, or stomachaches.

g. You may lose interest in sex.

You and your partner may react to diabetes in very different ways. The following exercises encourage both of you to look at how each of you thinks and feels about diabetes. Write your numeric answers on separate sheets. When finished, add up your scores and discuss your answers.

Quiz A —FOR THOSE WITH DIABETES

How do you feel about your diabetes?

0=never

1=sometimes

2=always

a. I feel angry because I have diabetes.

b. I feel stressed out about diabetes.

c. My diabetes is so overwhelming that I'd rather not deal with it.

d. I feel guilty about getting diabetes; it's probably my fault.

e. I feel depressed about diabetes.

f. I feel confused about how I'm supposed to treat my diabetes.

g. I'm frustrated because I can't seem to meet my diabetes goals.

h. I'm upset because I can't lose any weight.

i. I'm scared that I'll get complications, like blindness, amputation, or kidney failure that requires dialysis.

j. I worry about low blood sugar reactions.

Quiz B— FOR THOSE WHO LOVE SOMEONE WITH DIABETES

How do you think your partner feels about his or her diabetes?

0=never

1=sometimes

2=always

a. My partner feels angry because he/she has diabetes.

b. My partner feels stressed out about diabetes.

c. My partner's diabetes is so overwhelming that he/she would   rather not deal with it.

d. My partner feels guilty about having diabetes;

he/she thinks it is his/her fault.

e. My partner feels depressed about diabetes.

f. My partner feels confused about how to treat his/her diabetes.

g. My partner is frustrated because he/she doesn't always meet his/her diabetes goals.

h. My partner is upset because the diabetes medication has caused him/her to gain weight.

i. My partner is afraid that he/she will develop complications, like blindness, amputation, or kidney failure that requires dialysis.

j. My partner worries about low blood sugar reactions.

Who had the higher score? Does your partner think you're more, or less, distressed than you actually are? How do you both feel about this? On which specific items do you differ the most? What surprised you the most?

Now look at diabetes from your partner's point of view.

Quiz C —FOR THOSE WITH DIABETES

How do you think your partner feels about your diabetes?

0=never

1=sometimes

2=always

a. My partner feels angry about my diabetes.

b. My partner feels angry because he/she thinks I don't pay enough attention to diabetes.

c. My partner feels angry because he/she thinks I pay too much attention to diabetes.

d. My partner resents it when our plans change to accommodate my diabetes.

e. My partner is angry because he/she doesn't think I appreciate his/her efforts to help me.

f. My partner is convinced that I'll get serious complications.

g. My partner worries that I'll have low blood sugar reactions, especially at night.

Quiz D— FOR THOSE WHO LOVE SOMEONE WITH DIABETES

How do you feel about your loved one's diabetes?

0=never

1=sometimes

2=always

a. I feel angry because he/she has diabetes.

b. I feel angry when he/she seems to ignore his/her diabetes needs.

c. I dislike focusing so much of our time on diabetes.

d. I resent it when our plans change to accommodate his/her diabetes.

e. I get angry when he/she doesn't appreciate my efforts to help.

f. I feel afraid that he/she will get complications.

g. I worry that he/she will have low blood sugar reactions, especially at night.

Add up your score for Quiz C or D and compare once again. Who had the higher score? Does your partner think you're more, or less, distressed than you actually are? How do you both feel about this? On which specific items do you differ the most? What surprised you the most? Given what you've learned, how can you support each other even better?

It is difficult to be a supportive friend and partner when difficult feelings aren't discussed. Identifying and sharing your feelings are just the beginning. Here are some ways to help address these emotions.

Don't Ignore Your Diabetes

If you ignore your diabetes, will your difficult emotions go away? Ignoring a problem that you can't change sometimes makes sense, but diabetes is different. You can influence the course of this disease. Over the long term, ignoring it will only hurt you emotionally and physically.

> I developed type 2 diabetes after giving birth to my son Thomas four years ago and I'm still angry about it. I try to ignore it, but when I deny myself a favorite dessert or extra helping of food, I feel so deprived. Then there are times when I do ignore it and eat those desserts.
>
> —Suzanne

Several years ago, researchers interviewed a group of 30 men who were hospitalized for serious heart problems. Surprisingly, the ones who recovered the fastest during their hospital stay were the patients who minimized the seriousness of their condition, verbalizing comments such as, "This won't affect my life very much," and "This is no big deal." By doing this, these gentlemen found a way to protect themselves emotionally, which positively influenced their initial healing rate. But then they went home.

Although these men initially recovered more quickly, they did less well over the long term. In the year following their hospitalization, they were less likely to make healthy lifestyle changes and in the end spent much more time back in the hospital. Don't ignore your diabetes. Give your diabetes the care and attention that it deserves.

Express Your Emotions

Mark has been trying to lose weight since he was diagnosed with type 2 diabetes earlier this year. When he gets on the scale he seems so disappointed. The dial barely moves—all that work and nothing to show for it. He doesn't say a word, but I can tell that he is terribly frustrated, and so am I. Every day he threatens to give up, which really scares me. I wish we could talk about this.

—Connie

Don't keep your feelings bottled up. It is perfectly fine to hate diabetes and to verbalize your emotions. Fortunately, diabetes is one of the few conditions that will improve if you give it proper attention.

Mickey developed type 2 diabetes about four years ago and ignored it. I was so angry at him. He never tested his blood, totally ignored his doctor's orders to exercise, and conveniently "lost" the diet that the dietitian created for him. He was no longer the Mickey that I had married—someone who loved to tackle any challenge. I finally decided to stop being angry at him and direct my anger at the real culprit—his diabetes. I called it "Camilla" after Camilla Parker Bowles, the woman who came between Prince Charles and Princess Diana. Our "Camilla" entered, uninvited, into our home. Doing this brought things into better perspective for me and added some laughter into our lives—Mark loved blaming everything on Camilla! I stopped nagging Mark, and removing that pressure got him motivated to change. He decided to start walking every day and now finds that he enjoys it. He even started to care about his food choices. Things are looking up.

—Joyce

Some of the feelings you have about diabetes may be based on misinformation. Learn all you can, then reexamine what you thought to be true. The more you know about this condition, the more confident and comfortable you'll feel. Attend educational conferences, subscribe to magazines, read books, and meet with healthcare professionals. We learn new things about diabetes every day. Try some of the newer treatments that can make life easier for you and help you develop a more positive attitude.

Treat Abnormal Glucose Levels

When blood sugar levels stay high, a person can feel down in the dumps and lethargic.

> I never know what to expect when Diane shows up for work at our law office. She has had type 1 diabetes since the age of 12. By now, you would think that she would have this whole thing under control. Instead, she is moody, tired, and cranky. Then she has a snack and suddenly becomes easygoing and nice. I can't predict which of her many personalities will show up when she walks into the office. We work very closely together, and I don't know what to do.
>
> —Kurt

Abnormal blood sugar levels often cause unpleasant mood swings. If your blood sugar alternates between being too high and too low, it can exhaust you and even promote feelings of depression. Fortunately, normalizing blood sugar levels may help raise your energy and can improve your mood. Discuss treatment options with your healthcare professional. New and more effective diabetes medications are being developed every day. It may be time to adjust your care plan so that you can enjoy improved control. If you continue to be depressed, seek help from a qualified mental health professional. Serious forms of depression don't go away just because blood sugar levels improve.

Take Care of Yourself

Working through difficult emotions can be stressful and exhausting. Find ways to keep yourself and your environment calm.

a. Share your frustrations with a friend, counselor, or member of the clergy.

b. Get a massage.

c. Go to the gym.

d. Get to bed early.

e. Meet a friend for lunch or coffee.

f. Take a walk.

g. Exercise.

h. See a movie.

i. Listen to your favorite music.

j. Enjoy a date night with one you love.

Acknowledging your feelings is just the first step. Discuss the following questions with your partner:

a. Do you or I feel that diabetes is harming our social life?

b. Does it seem that diabetes is messing up our future dreams? How so?

c. Does it sometimes feel like diabetes dominates our lives?

d. Do you or I feel that my condition is hopeless?

Here are our thoughts on each of these questions:

Does diabetes affect your social life?

It doesn't have to! Don't allow diabetes to dominate your schedule. Plan ahead to make sure that your needs are met, then enjoy yourself. Seek out tools and treatments that make diabetes less of a burden. If you hate taking shots, try a pen or insulin pump. If you dislike food restrictions, explore alternate approaches to meal planning. Don't let diabetes rob you of the important moments of your life.

Does diabetes interfere with your future dreams?

We all expect to be healthy for many years, but sometimes illness makes an unannounced appearance. Don't allow diabetes to deter you from your dreams. Individuals with diabetes fly planes, work at high-level positions in corporations, run for public office, participate in the Olympics, appear on television, climb mountains, run marathons, have children, and do everything that people without diabetes do. Take care of your diabetes and many of your dreams will come true.

Does diabetes dominate your lives?

Every waking moment does not have to revolve around diabetes. You can have the life that you have always dreamed of. It may take a bit more effort, but it can be done.

> I always felt like a slave to my diabetes. I had to think of it before anything else. I was constantly afraid of making a mistake; a wrong piece of food or incorrect dose of medication could set me up for a fall. Then I took the diabetes class at my local hospital. The teacher was this delightful woman, Jane, from England. She corrected a lot of the misunderstandings that I had about diabetes and helped me create a reasonable care plan. I now feel that I control my diabetes, and not the other way around.
>
> —Lynn

Do you feel that your condition is hopeless?

Diabetes complications are not inevitable. Good diabetes control can slow down the development of complications or even help you avoid them altogether. With new tools and technology now available to us, we know that with effort and attention you can live a long and healthy life. If you see a healthcare provider who is not supportive, seek out one who is. You deserve the best life possible, and you can have it. Diabetes does not have to keep you down.

Depression and Diabetes

Serious forms of depression are common in people who have diabetes. Those who become depressed may feel less motivated to check their blood, exercise, take medication, or even eat. This sets off a downward spiral that is difficult to stop and can become life threatening.

No quiz can formally diagnose depression. But this modified version of the CES-D (Center for Epidemiological Studies-Depression) Scale, a widely used tool for depression screening, can give you an idea of how depressed you may be and if you should seek the help of a mental health professional.

On a piece of paper, write down the number that best describes how often you felt or behaved the ways listed during the past week:

0=Rarely or none of the time (less than once a day)

1=Occasionally or a little of the time (1–2 days)

2=Some of the time (3–4 days)

3=All of the time (5–7 days)

a. I was bothered by things that usually don't bother me.

b. I did not feel like eating; my appetite was poor.

c.   I felt that I could not shake off the blues even with help from my family and friends.

d.   I felt that I was just not as good as other people.

e.   I had trouble keeping my mind on what I was doing.

f.   I felt depressed.

g.   I felt that everything I did was an effort.

h.   I did not feel hopeful about the future.

i.   I thought my life had been a failure.

j.   I felt fearful.

k.   My sleep was restless.

l.   I was unhappy.

m. I talked less than usual.

n.   I felt lonely.

o.   I felt people were unfriendly.

p.   I did not enjoy life.

q.   I had crying spells.

r.   I felt sad.

s.   I felt that people disliked me.

t.   I could not get going.

If your total is 16 or higher, you may be suffering from depression, which can also affect your ability to manage your diabetes. Speak with your physician or meet with a mental health professional to evaluate the problem more thoroughly. For those who are clinically depressed, there are medications and forms of counseling that can help you get back on track.

If your total is less than 16, it is less likely that you have a serious form of depression. However, if you find these feelings troubling, don't ignore them. Talk to your physician and share your concerns with your loved ones.

Each person is unique, but for most individuals, depression results from a combination of factors that include your physical condition, the stresses in your world, and how you approach these stresses. A family history of depression raises your risk. Hormonal changes may contribute to depression, as can a variety of prescription medications.

Job loss, family stresses, death of a loved one, feelings of loneliness, and even early childhood trauma all increase the probability that depression may make an appearance in your life. How you view yourself in your world also makes a difference. If you tend to feel helpless and hopeless when confronted with life stresses, such as diabetes, your risk for depression climbs. Ask a member of your healthcare team to recommend a qualified mental health professional. He or she can help identify the causes of your symptoms and recommend effective treatment.

WHAT A PERSON WITH DIABETES MAY WANT HIS OR HER FRIENDS TO KNOW

1. I hate to admit it, but I can't always control my feelings, especially if my blood sugars are out of range.

2. I am not always open to advice from my loved ones. Sometimes I prefer to figure it out myself or get guidance exclusively from my healthcare team.

3. When aggravated or upset, I sometimes say things that I don't mean. If I do that, please know that I am sorry.

4. I really hate having diabetes!

WHAT A LOVED ONE MAY WANT THE PERSON WITH DIABETES TO KNOW

1. It is sometimes difficult to know the right thing to say or do when you are stressed or depressed about diabetes. Please don't be angry if I do or say the wrong thing.

2. I want to do the right thing and say the right words. I might not be successful, but I am trying.

3. I really hate diabetes, too!

When hard-to-deal-with diabetes emotions enter your relationships, they can affect them in profound ways. Discuss these issues with your loved ones. Don't let negative feelings fester. Seek out professional counseling assistance if the situation fails to improve. Diabetes can be overwhelming, but it doesn't have to ruin your relationships. Don't let it.

Chapter 5

Don't Be a Diabetes
Couch Potato

Do you want to be more motivated to care for your diabetes but need a push? It's a "Catch 22." First, you neglect your diabetes care, which leads to chronically high blood sugar levels. Then, your high blood sugar leaves you fatigued, edgy, angry, uncomfortable, depressed, and even less motivated. If you have loved ones who care about you, your less-than-perfect effort is probably driving them crazy.

But wait—what if you are doing well and don't know it? It may sound ridiculous, but it is a real possibility. Your A1C test will tell you if it's so.

Is Your A1C, A-OK?

A hemoglobin A1C is one of the best ways to assess your diabetes control. It is a simple blood test that measures your average blood sugar levels for the past two to three months. Here's how it works: The hemoglobin in your red blood cells carries oxygen to the cells of your body. When excess blood glucose enters the red blood cells, the hemoglobin becomes "glycated," or attached, to the glucose: the more glucose in your blood, the greater the amount of glycated hemoglobin.

When your blood sugar levels are close to normal for several months, your red blood cells look a bit like corn flakes. In the presence of chronically high glucose levels, they resemble sugar-frosted flakes. The A1C test measures how "sugar frosted" your blood cells are. Glycated ("sugar frosted") hemoglobin stays in the blood stream for two to three months.

To understand your A1C result, compare it to its blood glucose equivalent. For example, an A1C of 7 percent is equivalent to an estimated average blood sugar range of approximately 150–170 mg/dl.

A1C level (%)	Estimated equivalent average blood sugar range	
	mg/dl*	mmol/L*
4	60–80	3.3–4.4
5	90–110	5–6.1
6	120–135	6.7–7.5
7	150–170	8.3–9.4
8	180–205	10–11.4
9	210–240	11.7–13.3
10	250–275	13.9–15.3
11	280–310	15.6–17.2
12	320–345	17.8–19.2
13	350–375	19.4–20.8

*plasma values

Mindy has type 2 diabetes and takes oral diabetes medication. Her family accuses her of ignoring her condition, but she disagrees. She exercises regularly and tries to eat right. When she checks her blood, which isn't that often, it is usually after lunch, and her blood glucose is about 200 mg/dl. Mindy is scared that her doctor will tell her to begin insulin therapy. But at her appointment, she receives a pleasant surprise: her A1C is under 7 percent, indicating that her overall control is pretty good.

The A1C is valuable because it is an average of all of your glucose results over an extended period of time. A blood glucose monitor offers a snapshot of your glucose levels at an exact moment. It doesn't provide information about other times of the day or night. You could, therefore, have great overall blood glucose control yet not know it if you check your blood on a random basis and have a few abnormal results. On the other hand, you could have acceptable home blood sugar test results but not realize that your overall control is poor. Let your A1C define your progress.

Most experts recommend an A1C goal of less than 7 percent. Some suggest a goal of under 6.5 percent. If your A1C meets either recommendation, then whatever you are doing is pretty darn good, though you still need to pay attention to your blood pressure and cholesterol levels, which are as important as your blood sugars. Pat yourself on the back, keep up the good work, and let your friends and family know that all is well.

Occasionally, an A1C value can be misleading. If you don't feel well most of the time, your blood glucose levels might be swinging to extremes throughout the day and night. Because the A1C is an average of these levels, frequent highs and lows will average out to a reasonable result. Check your blood sugar level at different times of the day, such as before and after meals and exercise, to see if you are "swinging." If so, speak with your healthcare provider, share a detailed account of your daily activity and eating schedule, and together decide what you can do to prevent future excessive highs and lows.

Everyone Wants to Be Healthy

Maintaining good diabetes control takes some effort. What if you are tired of exercising, checking blood sugar levels, monitoring food portions, going to appointments, and inspecting your feet?

I've had type 2 for about two years. I know that I should exercise, eat healthy, and lose weight, but I hate the whole thing. Worst of all, my doctor just told me that he is giving up on me! To top it off, my husband and son think that yelling at me will motivate me into action. On the contrary, I do even less when they yell, just to teach them a lesson. I sound like a baby, I know. I have to do something about this, but I'm sick of the whole thing.

—Teresa

We all want to feel good and be healthy, but lethargy and temptations can get the best of us. Let's take physical activity. Last night you planned to exercise. You had every intention of doing it but got caught up in the newest television reality show, and before you knew it, the evening was gone. To make healthier choices, try to understand the personal pressures that prevent you from choosing the better options—the ones that help you control your diabetes.

What might prevent you from doing all that you can to control your diabetes?

1. *A lack of information.* If you don't understand diabetes, it will be difficult to treat it and difficult to improve your control. Attending classes, reading, and asking questions can really help.

2. *A lack of skills.* Can you use a blood glucose monitor correctly? Do you know how to count carbohydrates or prepare a diabetes-friendly meal? Diabetes requires a new set of skills that are needed to perform important care activities. Ask members of your healthcare team to help you learn the needed skills.

3. *A lack of confidence.* Diabetes changes over time. What works for you today may not work a year or two from now. When this happens, it is easy to blame yourself and lose confidence in your ability to manage your diabetes. You must continue to learn and implement new care techniques.

4. *The belief that you've already lost the war.* You've cut back on your food portions and increased your exercise, but when you climb onto the scale, it displays the same weight as last week.

That is frustrating, but don't despair: you are probably improving. Muscle weighs more than fat, so as you develop new muscle from your increased physical activity, forget the scale. Instead, monitor how your clothes fit and note the inches that you lose on your waist, thighs, and biceps to track your progress. Additional muscle burns calories while you are at rest, so your weight loss efforts will continue after you shower and change. Your blood sugar levels should also improve with the healthy lifestyle changes that you are making, and that will let you control your diabetes with less medication.

5. *Possible depression.* People with diabetes are at a higher risk for developing a depressive illness than other individuals. If depressed, you will have a difficult time doing many positive healthcare tasks. Effective treatments for depression are available. Ask your healthcare professionals about them.

6. *The belief that your diabetes is not so serious.* Some people think that their diabetes is not serious, especially if they feel fine or don't need to take insulin. Don't ignore your diabetes. All types are very serious and can become deadly if ignored. A patient with type 2 once compared her diabetes to an animal:

> If you treat your diabetes right, it will crawl into the corner and fall asleep. If you ignore it, it will wake up and make a heck of a lot of trouble!
>
> —Brenda

Take Control of Your Diabetes

There are many ways to get yourself off the couch to care for your diabetes. Think about the people you love and the things you value:

a. Your spouse. You want to share a full and healthy life together.

b. Your children. You want to be there for them as they grow up.

c. Your dreams. You want to enjoy living them.

d. Your goals. You want to finish the projects and plans that you've started.

e. Your health. Well-controlled diabetes slows down or helps prevent the development of diabetes complications. With good care, you should be able to live a long and healthy life with diabetes.

You control your diabetes, no one else. Your doctor doesn't live with you and your dietitian is not on the way over to cook dinner. Even loved ones have their own issues on their minds. No one can force you to care for your illness. Your diabetes is yours and yours alone. To improve your control, know what you are doing. Have you attended a diabetes education program? Have you had your questions answered by knowledgeable experts? Do you know what you are supposed to do? Have you had your A1C, blood pressure, and cholesterol levels checked recently? Do you know what your results mean? If so, you are well on your way. Now set small, realistic goals.

Terri has had type 2 diabetes for 12 years. She needs to lose weight but has failed at every weight loss attempt she has ever tried. She finally took her doctor's advice and made an appointment to meet with a registered dietitian who specializes in diabetes.

Terri: I'd like to lose 50 pounds by my birthday, which is at the end of this month. Is that unreasonable?

Dietitian: Yes, Terri, a weight loss goal of more than a pound each day is unreasonable and unsafe. An average weight loss in a healthy weight-reduction program is one or two pounds per week! You won't succeed if your expectations are unrealistic, and they will undermine any motivation that you have scraped together. Small, realistic steps combined with frequent rewards will help keep you focused on your goals.

Lance consistently meets his weight-loss goals and keeps his enthusiasm high. How does he do it?

I have type 2 diabetes and I'd like to lose 70 pounds more to lower my insulin resistance and reduce my need for medication. Seventy pounds is too overwhelming, so I just ignore it. Instead, I focus on a weight loss goal of two pounds. It may take me a week or so, but I can handle that goal. I eat healthy foods in reasonable portions, do some physical activity each day, and drink a glass of water before each meal and snack. When the scale goes down, I smile the entire day. I feel great. When I meet that goal, I give myself a day to enjoy the accomplishment, then hit the treadmill and go for another two pounds.

Your Inner Voice

We each have a tiny voice that speaks to us. It calls to us when we see scoops of delicious mint chocolate-chip ice cream swimming in hot fudge, nuts, and whipped cream, all topped with a cherry.

Your Inner Voice: Hey, no one is looking. You deserve some ice cream. You've had a hard day. Come on!

You: No, I'm not going to do it. My blood sugar will soar.

Between the two voices, who is going to win?

For many people, the gooey sundae will win hands down unless they can quiet their devilish inner voice. Short-term gains usually win over long-term benefits. Conversations like the one above can steer you off course. Set realistic goals to help silence that inner voice.

Goal #1: Stay away from the ice cream shop for two weeks. Try reduced-calorie, sugar-free frozen desserts instead, like artificially sweetened fudge pops.

Goal #2: If all goes well, extend Goal #1 for an additional two weeks. If you can't meet this goal, attempt one that is easier to meet. Perhaps one week. Or even one day at a time. Build on each success, step by step.

Caring for diabetes is not always easy. To succeed, you must be able to adapt your goals to your lifestyle:

> I have had type 2 diabetes for four years. I was doing great. I walked each morning, came home, got ready for work and then had a great day. But I just got promoted, and now I have to head for the office much earlier. My exercise schedule doesn't work for me anymore. I don't have enough time to shower and change, so I stopped exercising altogether. I should find another time but haven't done so yet.
>
> —Lucy

A schedule change, like Lucy's, can throw off a finely tuned activity program. If you were doing well, regroup. Remind yourself of the value of your efforts and reschedule them back into your life. It is common to meet a person who "used to" walk on the beach every day. Most folks "used to" do a lot of healthy things but stopped when their lives changed. Take control of your life. Personal trainer Sean Robbins likes to say: "Invest in your body. It's the most important stock you will ever have." Of course, it may not be easy to do. Like Lucy, you might be overwhelmed with other tasks. Sometimes it takes a bit of thought to get what you need.

Lucy solved her situation in this way:

I asked around. It turns out that there is a workout room on a lower floor in our office building, which several co-workers use during lunch. I decided to join them. I now get my physical activity in every day and have made a few new friends.

Rating Your Readiness

Now that you're charged up, let's find the barriers that keep you from meeting your diabetes goals. It is one thing to set reasonable goals but a whole other thing to achieve them. The following exercise assesses your readiness to begin an activity. If you aren't ready, it will help you discover why and offer ways to get over the roadblocks.

List several activities that you would like to begin in order to improve your diabetes. Be specific and make each choice measurable. "I'd like to swim more" is too vague. Instead, write "Swim 4 times a week for at least 20 minutes."

Georgia has type 1 diabetes. She asked her husband Ronnie to do this exercise with her. Here are the measurable actions Georgia listed to help control her diabetes. Ronnie made his personal health list as well:

Georgia's List:

1. Walk 5 times a week for at least 20 minutes.

2. Inspect my feet for cuts, bruises, and red areas before bed.

3. Check my blood sugar twice a day—once in the morning and two hours after dinner.

Ronnie's List:

1. Ride my bike for at least 30 minutes, or do an equivalent activity, 5 times each week.

2. Eat at least one vegetable or drink tomato juice at every meal.

3. Get to sleep before 11:00 p.m.

Now, list a few of the healthy actions that you would like to begin. Be specific and make each activity measurable.

Next, rate your choices. Be honest. You have healthy and wonderful goals, but how ready are you to do them? Here is how Georgia evaluated her list. She rated her goals on a scale of 1 to 5.

5 = I'm very ready. I'm starting tomorrow!

4 = I'm almost there. I'll start this weekend.

3 = I'll begin in two weeks.

2 = I'll start next month.

1 = I'm not ready.

Georgia's Health Activities	*Her Readiness Rating*
1. Walk 5 times a week.	5

Georgia is psyched! She has her walking shoes and plans to begin first thing tomorrow morning. She likes walking but never made time for it. Now that she has committed to it, she is excited and ready to begin. Georgia plans to call her neighbor to ask her to join her. She knows that it is harder to cancel a workout when someone counts on you to show up. Besides, it makes the walk more fun!

2. Inspect my feet before bed.	5

This is easy to do. Georgia met with her podiatrist to review the proper way to inspect her feet. She plans to do this each night before going to bed.

3. Check my blood sugar twice a day.	2

Georgia is not ready to do this last task and needs to consider the questions below. If any of your actions have a readiness rating that is less than 4, answer the following:

1. Why is this activity important to your diabetes health?

2. Why did you rank it less than 5?

3. What can you do to raise its readiness rating?

4. Is there a way for your partner to help you with this task?

Here are Georgia's responses:

1. Why is this activity important to your diabetes health?

"I know that checking my blood is the best way for me to monitor my diabetes progress."

2. Why did you rank it less than 5?

"It hurts! I hate doing it. It takes time and is annoying."

3. What can you do to raise its readiness rating?

"Instead of twice a day, I will check my blood sugar once a day. I can do that. I'd also like to see the effect that my daily walks have on my blood sugar levels. That interests me. Finally, I'm going to buy a glucose monitor that does alternate site tests. I'm sick of taking blood from my fingers and could take blood from my forearm and other locations. I'd like that."

4. Is there a way for your partner to help you with this task?

"I'd like to have my husband sit by me when I take my blood. I get really squeamish and would love to have him nearby."

Now rate your own activity readiness, using the same format shown above.

> 5 = I'm very ready. I'm starting tomorrow!
>
> 4 = I'm almost there. I'll start this weekend.
>
> 3 = I'll begin in two weeks.
>
> 2 = I'll start next month.
>
> 1 = I'm not ready.

If any of your actions have readiness ratings less than 4, answer these questions:

1. Why is this activity important to your diabetes health?
2. Why did you rank it less than 4?
3. What can you do to raise its readiness rating?
4. Is there a way for your partner to help you with this task?

Setting healthy goals is important for everyone. Help your partner evaluate his or her activity choices in the same way.

WHAT A PERSON WITH DIABETES MAY WANT HIS OR HER FRIENDS TO KNOW

1. I know what to do to control my diabetes, but that doesn't mean that I am ready to do it. I sometimes need time to get motivated.
2. I sometimes enjoy working out with someone.
3. I get frustrated with myself when I don't care for my diabetes.

WHAT A LOVED ONE MAY WANT THE PERSON WITH DIABETES TO KNOW

1. I often get frustrated when I see you neglect your diabetes care.

2. I get scared when I think of the complications that may develop when you ignore your diabetes care.

3. I need to understand how difficult it is for you to stick to your goals. If you have to make quality food choices, then I will too. If you have to exercise, then I will do it also. We will both benefit.

Chapter 6

Is It Time to Panic?

What is a diabetes emergency? When is the right time to run, drop everything, and get immediate assistance? Surprisingly, very few situations are actual emergencies and most can be dealt with calmly. Stress will rein supreme if:

a. You panic unnecessarily.

b. You and your loved ones disagree on whether a situation is an emergency or not.

c. You and your loved ones can't agree on what to do when a challenging moment arrives.

Learn the truth about these situations, gain confidence in dealing with them, and relax.

> I love my wife so much. I worry that she will have a sudden drop in blood sugar, stop breathing, and leave me—right here, in the middle of the night. I get very little sleep these days.
> —Max

Max and Lorraine have been married for over 50 years. Lorraine developed type 1 diabetes in her 40s and now, at age 72, her blood sugar swings have become frequent and unexpected. Each night, Max sets his alarm clock for 3:00 a.m. so he can lovingly check on his wife as she sleeps. His nightly routine is exhausting, but he can't help it. It is something he feels compelled to do. Emergencies can happen, but in this case, Max, like many loved ones, is overreacting to a concern that deserves a calmer approach.

"I've been treating people with diabetes for over 20 years. I'm still waiting for the first real emergency of my career," says Steve, one of our authors.

Do diabetes emergencies really exist? Learn how to accurately assess the seriousness of a surprise diabetes event with only a little information and planning.

Not all diabetes situations are worth getting frantic about. Common diabetes crises fall into two categories: 1) emergencies that require you to drop everything and run for assistance; and 2) "urgencies" that deserve attention, yet do not need an immediate response.

> Audrey and Jerry grabbed their coats and quickly walked to the nearest exit at their favorite restaurant. Jerry had ordered a diet beverage and was sure that the waiter had brought him a regular Coke, which he consumed without thinking. They didn't know what to expect but were certain that it wouldn't be a pretty sight and wanted to be home so they could call the doctor, if needed.
>
> When they finally arrived home, Jerry was relieved. He checked his blood glucose level and found that it was fine. Audrey, on the other hand, was furious. Their lovely evening had again been cut short because of Jerry's diabetes.

Did Audrey and Jerry overreact? Yes. Could this situation (and the fight that followed) be avoided? Yes, this was not a true emergency. They need to learn how to calmly handle suspected high blood sugar levels. Have you ever misjudged a diabetes situation?

Below is an exercise that can help you put diabetes events into proper perspective. Answer yes or no to each of the following challenges. Take this quiz with your main diabetes-support partner. Each of you can write your answers on separate sheets of paper. Then check against the answers—and explanations—that follow.

Yes = Tend to this right now. Don't delay.

　　or

No = It's just an urgency. Tend to it soon, but don't drop everything to seek immediate help.

1. Your blood sugar rises above 300 mg/dl (16.7 mmol/L).
　　Yes or No

2. You have tingling in your feet.
　　Yes or No

3. Your doctor's office calls to say that you have protein in your urine.
　　Yes or No

4. You feel a tightness in your chest for several minutes on multiple occasions.
　　Yes or No

5. For the first time ever, you cannot get or maintain an erection.
　　Yes or No

6. Your blood sugar is 39 mg/dl (2.2 mmol/L), yet you feel fine.
　　Yes or No

7. You forget to take a dose of insulin.
　　Yes or No

8. You mistake your long-acting insulin for your fast-acting and take the wrong one.
　　Yes or No

9. You accidentally double your dose of insulin.
   Yes or No

10. You accidentally take an extra diabetes pill.
    Yes or No

11. You go to bed and forget to take your long-acting insulin.
    Yes or No

12. Your partner notices that you don't respond to comments made by others and are drooling.
    Yes or No

13. You have the flu for several days, accompanied by uncontrolled vomiting and blood sugars of over 300 mg/dl (16.7 mmol/L).
    Yes or No

14. You wake up and have swollen ankles.
    Yes or No

15. You eat a giant piece of gooey chocolate layer cake, by accident, of course.
    Yes or No

Here are the correct answers:

1. Your blood sugar rises above 300 mg/dl (16.7 mmol/L).
   No, it's just an urgency.

2. You have tingling in your feet.
   No, it's just an urgency.

3. Your doctor's office calls to say that you have protein in your urine.
   No, it's just an urgency.

4. You feel a tightness in your chest for several minutes on multiple occasions.

      Yes, tend to this now.

5. For the first time ever, you cannot get or maintain an erection.

      No, it's just an urgency.

6. Your blood sugar is 39 mg/dl (2.2 mmol/L), yet you feel fine.

      Yes, tend to this now.

7. You forget to take a dose of mealtime insulin.

      Yes, tend to this now.

8. You mistake your long-acting insulin for your fast-acting and take the wrong one.

      Yes, tend to this now.

9. You accidentally double your dose of insulin.

      Yes, tend to this now.

10. You accidentally take an extra diabetes pill.

      Yes, tend to this now.

11. You go to bed and forget to take your long-acting insulin.

      No, it's just an urgency.

12. Your partner notices that you don't respond to comments made by others and are drooling.

      Yes, tend to this now.

13. You have the flu for several days, accompanied by uncontrolled vomiting and blood sugars of over 300 mg/dl (16.7 mmol/L).

      Yes, tend to this now.

14. You wake up and have swollen ankles.

      Yes, tend to this now.

15. You eat a giant piece of gooey chocolate layer cake.
    No, it's just an urgency.

How well did you both do? Now, let's see why these events are classified either as emergencies or urgencies.

1. Your blood sugar rises above 300 mg/dl (16.7 mmol/L).

Abnormally high blood sugar levels are almost never serious emergencies. Why? Even though high blood glucose levels are not healthy, it is possible to function quite well at an extremely elevated level for a brief period of time, even up to several days, as long as you don't become dehydrated. It is not recommended, but it can be done. Here are suggested ways to deal with this situation. If you wish, share them with your partner, friends, and family members to keep them informed if this situation arises.

If you take oral diabetes medication only, try these treatment ideas:

a. Monitor your blood sugar every two hours.

b. Drink plenty of sugar-free fluids, including water.

c. Go for a gentle walk. Vigorous exercise is not recommended and could worsen the situation by encouraging your blood glucose level to climb further.

d. Skip or delay your next meal, or eliminate any fast-acting carbohydrates that you planned to eat, like fruits and fruit juices.

If you use insulin, try these strategies:

a. Delay your next meal.

b. Eat less than your planned amount of food.

c. Eliminate or replace foods that contain quick-acting sugars, such as fruit juice.

d. Replace milk or any calorie-containing beverage with a non-caloric one.

e. At your next meal, increase the time delay between eating and your insulin shot.

f. Do not finish your next meal, but spread the remaining calories throughout the entire day. For example, save your bagel or apple for later.

g. Do gentle exercise after eating. A slow leisurely stroll is a good choice. Avoid strenuous exercise, which can elevate your blood sugar further.

h. If high blood sugar events occur frequently, work with your healthcare team to adjust your diabetes care plan, or make your own changes if you know how to do this.

i. Some of you may need additional insulin to normalize your blood glucose levels. Use your personal "correction factor" to estimate the amount your blood sugar levels should go down when you take 1 unit of fast-acting insulin.

Your Insulin Correction Factor

Here is one of the many ways to compute your insulin correction factor:

a. Estimate how many units of insulin you use in an average day.

b. Divide 1500 by your total daily units. (Some use 1800.)

c. The answer is your correction factor (CF), which is the approximate amount that your blood sugar should drop when you take 1 unit of insulin.

Here is how Sue estimated her CF:

a. Sue uses about 30 units of insulin each day.

b. 1500 divided by 30 = 50 (her correction factor)

c. One unit of insulin should drop her blood sugar by about 50 mg/dl.

A possible scenario would go like this. Sue's blood sugar is 250 mg/dl. Her target level is 100 mg/dl. She subtracts her target level from her current level:

$$\begin{array}{r} 250 \text{ (current level)} \\ -100 \text{ (desired level)} \\ \hline 150 \text{ mg/dl} \end{array}$$

She needs to reduce her blood sugar level by 150 mg/dl. Her correction factor is 50. If 1 unit of insulin will lower her blood sugar by 50 mg/dl, then Sue needs to take 3 units of insulin.

To determine your own correction factor, simply divide 1500 by the number of insulin units you use each day. If you use mmol/L, divide 83 by your total daily insulin units (some use 100 instead of 83). Keep this figure handy to control unexpected spikes in your blood sugar level.

It takes a while for blood sugar to come down, so be patient. Fast-acting insulin stays active in the body for about four hours; it needs time to act. Check your blood sugar level every two hours to be sure that it is going down, but don't take additional insulin until four hours have passed.

Extremely high blood sugar levels—over 300 mg/dl (16.7 mmol/L)—are often tolerated differently by those with type 1 and type 2. People with type 1 can usually handle a high blood sugar level for quite a while. For those with type 2, an extremely high blood sugar level can be troublesome and become dangerous if accompanied by severe dehydration.

2. You have tingling in your feet.

Tingling is not an emergency but may be an early sign of diabetes nerve damage (neuropathy), which progresses very slowly. The type of neuropathy seen in diabetes usually starts in both feet. If this problem persists, make an appointment with a podiatrist. If your symptoms are due to diabetes, you have probably caught it early enough to prevent it from progressing.

3. Your doctor's office calls to say that you have protein in your urine.

Small amounts of protein in your urine (microalbuminuria) may be a sign that your kidneys require attention, but this is not an emergency. It takes five to eight years before the condition evolves to the point where dangerously large amounts of protein appear. A variety of problems can cause this to happen, such as diabetic retinopathy (eye disease), high cholesterol levels, heart disease, or even strenuous exercise. It is not necessarily the result of kidney disease.

A positive protein test should be confirmed by an additional test before beginning aggressive therapy. A lot can be done to prevent diabetes kidney disease from progressing, including improved glucose control, blood pressure control, various medications and a low-protein meal plan. Relax and meet with your doctor.

4. You feel a tightness in your chest for several minutes on multiple occasions.

You may be having a heart attack and should get assistance immediately. Heart disease is the number one killer of eight out of every ten individuals with diabetes. A heart attack happens when a blockage reduces blood flow to the heart, depriving it of needed oxygen for a long period of time and causing damage to the heart muscles.

Fortunately, there is a life-saving treatment. Streptokinase, a powerful substance, can be infused into the blocked artery to dissolve the clot and help the blood flow more freely. For this drug to be effective, it must be given within four hours of the first sensation of pain. Other symptoms of a heart attack are shortness of breath, weakness, fainting, abdominal pain, and dizziness. If you believe that you are having a heart attack, drop everything and go to the nearest emergency room for assistance. This is an emergency.

5. For the first time ever, you cannot get or maintain an erection.

This is upsetting for you and your partner, but it is no cause for panic. It is extremely common for a man to occasionally have difficulty getting or maintaining an erection, even without diabetes. This does not mean that a serious medical condition is developing. See Chapter 10 for more on this.

6. Your blood sugar is 39 mg/dl (2.2 mmol/L), yet you feel fine.

A low blood sugar level can be serious and should be treated right away. First recheck your blood glucose result. Most meters have a 10–15 percent error rate and may be off as much as 20 percent if the reading is extremely high or low.

The most common symptoms of low blood sugar are sweating, shaking, a feeling that your heart is racing, and confusion. A person could also feel perfectly fine, yet still have a dangerously low blood sugar level. The most common causes of hypoglycemia (low blood sugar) are too much insulin or diabetes medication, too little food, or excessive physical activity.

Fortunately, serious low blood sugar events are not as common as some believe them to be. If you have type 1, you might experience mild hypoglycemia when you adjust your insulin dose, change your food choices, or increase physical activity. If you have type 2 and control it with diet and exercise, a severe low blood sugar episode will be rare, and may never happen. A recent study published in *Diabetes Care* (2003), one of the premier journals for diabetes specialists, studied the prevalence of hypoglycemic episodes in individuals with diabetes:

Total number of people with diabetes studied: 8,655

Length of time of study: 12 months

Total number who had severe episodes of low blood sugar: 160, or less than 2%

Most people with diabetes rarely have life-threatening blood sugar lows. But if you are concerned, remember the "15 Rule" for treating hypoglycemia:

The 15 Rule

a. Eat 15 grams of a fast-acting carbohydrate, such as 4 ounces of fruit juice, 1 can of regular soda, 2 teaspoons of sugar, or commercially sold glucose tablets.

b. Wait 15 minutes and try not to panic.

c. Test again.

d. Repeat until you are within your target range or above 70mg/dl. If friends see that you can't swallow, they shouldn't attempt to feed you for fear of choking.

Instead, they should administer a shot of glucagon, which is explained further in scenario #12 below.

Don't use chocolate to treat low blood sugar events. It contains fat, can slow down the rise of glucose levels, and causes unwanted weight gain.

Admittedly, many folks find following this treatment for low blood sugar a challenge. The unpleasant feelings of shakiness, sweating, headache, fatigue, etc., often throw people into a panic, and they frantically gulp down anything in sight to alleviate these feelings. Do not eat and eat until these uncomfortable symptoms disappear. Stop snacking once your blood glucose levels get to a safe level—above 70 mg/dl (3.9 mmol/L).

The unpleasant symptoms that accompany hypoglycemia improve slowly, sometimes quite a while after the body's blood sugar levels have returned to normal. If you experience frequent bouts of hypoglycemia, meet with your health care team to adjust your diabetes regimen. Until then the 15 Rule is the way to go.

7. You forget to take a dose of mealtime insulin.

Don't panic but take immediate action. The concern here is time. How long have you been without insulin? Have you gone so long that emergency steps are needed to normalize your glucose levels?

First, check your blood sugar. If you are within a normal range or are slightly high, relax and take the dose that you missed.

If you are above 300 mg/dl (16.7 mmol/L), take a correction dose of insulin and try the suggestions discussed in scenario #1 (above). Do not take the dose that you missed, only the correction amount. These actions will encourage your levels to return to normal.

8. You mistake your long-acting insulin for your fast-acting and take the long-acting dose.

You have taken additional insulin, and it's going to last a long time. Keep a close watch on your blood sugars throughout the day:

a. Check your blood sugar levels every 2–3 hours if you are greater than 200 mg/dl (11.1 mmol/L).

b. Check every hour if you are below 200 mg/dl. Most long-acting insulin remains active in your body for about 24 hours.

c. Set your alarm to wake up every 2–3 hours to make sure that you are in a safe range during the night.

d. Take snacks as needed. Use the 15 Rule instructions (see #6 above) to treat low blood sugar levels.

e. Turn this mishap into a positive. If you need a huge snack to bring your blood sugar levels up, now's the time to have that hot fudge sundae!

9. You accidentally double your dose of insulin.

This requires action. The type of insulin that you have taken will affect how you deal with it. If you have taken a double dose of long-acting insulin, see scenario #8 (above) for treatment options. If you have taken additional fast-acting insulin, monitor your blood sugar levels often over the next four hours or so.

If you count carbohydrates, total up the amount of insulin that you have taken and measure out an appropriate amount of carbohydrates to eat. If you are not familiar with that technique, eat double what you planned to consume and monitor your blood sugar levels for the next several hours. Treat lows as recommended in scenario #6 (above).

10. You accidentally take an extra diabetes pill.

No need to panic. Most oral medications take a while before they become effective. Fast-acting pills can take effect within 20 minutes, but most others need at least an hour. Check your blood sugar at regular intervals over the next several hours, and eat snacks if your levels drop below your target range. Use the 15 Rule (see scenario #6, above) to help you time your foods appropriately.

If you do not monitor your blood sugar levels, a practice often ignored by those with type 2 diabetes, now is a great time to start. Purchase a glucose monitor. If you don't feel well, have someone purchase one for you.

11. You go to bed and forget to take your long-acting insulin.

You can handle this. Long-acting insulin has that name because it lasts a very l-o-n-g t-i-m-e. You will wake up with an elevated blood sugar level, but don't panic. Take half of your nighttime insulin amount at that time, then your usual dose at bedtime. If you use fast-acting insulin, take small amounts of it during the day to treat elevated blood sugar levels.

12. Your partner notices that you don't respond to comments from others and are drooling.

He or she should take immediate action and keep a cool head. Your blood sugar level is dangerously low. If you cannot swallow safely, you can be treated quickly with a shot of glucagon. This substance raises blood glucose levels within 5–20 minutes. Ask your doctor if it is appropriate for you to keep a glucagon emergency kit in your household, at work, or in another location. If so, he or she will provide instructions on using it.

Review this information with those close to you. They should learn how to prepare the injection and how to check your blood sugar levels in order to monitor your response. People respond to glucagon very quickly. If no glucagon kit is handy and you are unable to swallow, have someone rub honey, glucose gel, syrup, or jelly on the inside of your mouth. Do not attempt to consume any type of food or drink. Call 911 for additional assistance.

13. You have the flu for several days, accompanied by uncontrolled vomiting and blood sugars of over 300 mg/dl (16.7 mmol/L).

Agree on your sick day plans long before any problem arises. This will help prevent a sick day from turning ugly. Post your plans prominently and review them with those close to you. Here are some guidelines:

Take your diabetes medication, even if you are not eating.

When illness strikes, the body becomes resistant to the blood-glucose-lowering effect of diabetes medications. Instead of cutting your meds out altogether, you may actually need additional amounts.

Check your blood often.

Monitor your blood glucose levels every 2–3 hours if you take insulin and 3–4 times per day if you have type 2 diabetes and take diabetic pills. Chapter 7 shows you how to interpret your glucose monitor results.

Drink lots of non-caloric, caffeine-free beverages.

Nausea, vomiting, and inadequate fluid intake can cause dehydration. Drink liberal amounts of water or liquids that are artificially sweetened and do not contain caffeine or sugar.

Take a correction dose of insulin, if needed.

If you take fast-acting insulin like Regular, Humalog, or Novolog, you may need to take small to medium doses throughout the day to prevent your blood sugar from going above 200 mg/dl (11.1 mmol/L). Use your insulin correction factor (see scenario #1, above) to determine the amount of insulin to use.

If you are vomiting, test for ketones.

Ketone bodies can appear in the urine if your illness becomes severe. They develop when the body breaks down fat instead of sugar as an energy source. This situation is dangerous as it can change the acid/base balance in your blood. To test for ketones, dip a specially prepared strip into a urine sample. Positive results will require you to monitor your blood glucose more closely, take additional amounts of insulin, or visit the emergency room.

14. You wake up and have swollen ankles.

Swollen ankles could be a symptom of heart failure, which can cause a buildup of fluids in the body's tissues. When blood leaving the heart slows down its pace, the blood returning to the heart through the veins backs up and causes swelling. Immediate help is needed if redness, a feeling of heat in your legs, pain, or shortness of breath accompanies the swelling. There are many causes of swollen ankles, some more serious than others. Even if the symptoms mentioned above don't appear, make an appointment with your healthcare provider to let him or her know that this is happening.

15. You eat a giant piece of gooey chocolate layer cake.

Check your blood glucose within 1–2 hours and treat high levels as suggested in scenario # 1, above, or as directed by your healthcare team. Your blood glucose levels may climb for a while, but a temporarily high level is not an emergency room type of situation. You can handle it.

How Well Did You Do?

Add up your correct answers and your partner's.

13–15 correct: Great. You know what to do.

10–12 correct: Not bad. Just review a bit more.

9 or less correct: Not good. Start reviewing now.

How do your answers compare with the explanations given above? Discuss the results with your partner.

1. How did you do?

2. Between the two of you, who had more correct answers?

3. Who had more incorrect answers? Which situations did you misjudge?

4. On how many items did you agree? Did you agree on how to handle these problems?

5. On how many did you disagree? Do you agree now since you have additional facts?

6. Did you consider most of the situations emergencies? If so, you may be overreacting to diabetes challenges. Worrying needlessly about potential diabetes problems is exhausting.

Agree on the role that each of you should play in any diabetes situation. The more prepared you are, the more confident and successful you will be.

Are You "Problem-Prone"?

It is easy to doubt your ability to manage your condition if you have frequent diabetes problems. Friends and relatives may lose confidence in you and start to view you as fragile or incompetent. Researchers at the University of Virginia Health Sciences Center in Charlottesville also found that frequent and severe low blood sugar episodes can negatively affect intimate relationships:

Spouses of patients with a recent history of severe hypoglycemia showed significantly more fear of hypoglycemia, mari-
tal conflict about diabetes management, and sleep distur-
bances caused by hypoglycemia.

—*Diabetes Care*, 1997

Learn all you can about diabetes from this book and
from other reliable sources listed in Suggested Resources at
the back of this book. Discuss the role that each of you
should play when problems arise. Knowing what to do and
when to do it will boost everyone's confidence. Plan ahead
before a difficult diabetes situation occurs.

Here is a sample action plan. Use the same headings
(shown in italics) to create an action plan of your own. Be
sure to have it approved by your healthcare team. Then discuss the plan with your loved ones and even with your coworkers. Let them know what to do if you have diabetes
needs that require help. Keep the plan handy, and let others
know where to find it.

Should you be prepared for unexpected diabetes
events? Sure. Should you drive yourself and others crazy worrying about them? No way.

Sue's Diabetes Action Plan

My Important Phone Numbers:

Doctor: Dr. Sugar (312) 555-1234
Diabetes Educator: Ms. Knowe (847) 555-5678
Podiatrist: Dr. Footsie (773) 555-2468
Pharmacy: Pills-R-Us (312) 555-3579

My Blood Sugar Goals:

Before breakfast: between 90–130 mg/dl
Before lunch: between 90–130 mg/dl
Two hours after the first bite of a meal: less than 160 mg/dl

At bedtime: between 110–150 mg/dl

A1C: less than 7%

When my blood sugar goes above my target range:

My correction factor is 50. I can take 1 unit of insulin to bring down my blood sugar by about 50 points. I will check my blood often. I will try walking and delay my next meal a bit. I can also skip or reduce the carbohydrates in my next meal.

When my blood sugar goes below my target range:

I will use the 15 Rule and check my blood sugar often. Some possible foods to eat to treat low blood sugar levels: cup juice, can regular soda (not diet), 2–5 glucose tablets.

It Ain't the Boy Scouts, But Always Be Prepared

Check your blood sugar levels before you get behind the wheel of a car, especially if you take insulin. Save your life and the lives of those around you, don't risk losing your license, and let your family know that you are safe behind the wheel.

Joan has type 1 diabetes and has been a diabetes educator for many years. She knows how to take care of her diabetes, but once in a while even experts get tripped up. One day she was rushed. Joan left work early to sign her son up for summer camp at the local community center. She parked her car several blocks away and ran to the office to get there before closing time. She started to sweat but blamed it on the hot Texas sun and her brisk pace. On her way home, the drama began:

I lost complete track of where I was. I knew something was wrong but couldn't think clearly enough to stop or get out glucose tablets. I gripped the wheel and desperately tried to stay in control of the car. I remember thinking, "God, I can't do this anymore." I let go of the wheel, rear-ended the car in front of me, and somehow managed to stop the car, though I don't recall exactly how. Two cars were totaled, but thank God, no one was hurt beyond my own split lip on the steering wheel. I lost my license for a year as "punishment."

Be sure that your blood sugar levels are within your normal range before you hit the road, and always keep fast-acting carbohydrate snacks in the car. If your levels are low, use the 15 Rule to get yourself back on track.

What if you forget your car snacks and are not near a store when your blood sugar drops? Pull over and use your cell phone to call for help. But remember, glucose tablets are portable, as are juice boxes and hard candies. Don't leave home without a snack in your pocket, purse, or glove compartment.

Low blood sugar is always dangerous for your body. But for most individuals with diabetes, it is rarely a life-threatening emergency. Here is a list of crisis supplies and suggested locations for storing them. Think of them as you do your household smoke alarm—it is there if you need it, but hopefully that time will never come.

The Car

> Fast-acting carbohydrate snacks like glucose tablets, juice boxes, and sugar packets
>
> Emergency contact information
>
> Blood glucose meter and supplies
>
> Snack foods for traffic delays, such as meal replacement bars or shakes, granola bars, nuts, crackers, etc.

The Office

> Foods to eat if a meal is delayed: crackers, nuts, cheese, and yogurt

Blood glucose meter and supplies

Diabetes pills, insulin pen

Fast-acting carbohydrate snacks stored in a clearly labeled drawer or box so coworkers can find them easily, if necessary

Emergency phone numbers

Pump supplies, if you are a pump wearer

The Gym Bag or Back Pack

Fast-acting carbohydrate snacks

Blood glucose meter and supplies

The Home

Fast-acting carbohydrate snacks

Emergency medical numbers

Juice boxes next to your bed for nighttime lows

Glucose monitors and supplies

Ketone strips in bathroom for sick days

Glucagon kit

WHAT A PERSON WITH DIABETES MAY WANT HIS OR HER FRIENDS TO KNOW

1. I get frustrated if my diabetes problems happen frequently. I must continuously fine-tune my treatment, which is a tough chore.

2. I need to keep diabetes supplies handy. I'd love your help in doing that.

3. I may not feel dangerous low blood-sugar symptoms. That happens with diabetes sometimes. Please let me know if you notice them.

4. I'd like to show you where I keep my emergency contact information and supplies.

5. Sometimes I can take care of diabetes problems all by myself.

6. Sometimes I can't take care of diabetes problems all by myself.

7. Let's agree on what to do before any challenging situations happen.

8. I'll stop saying "I'm fine" if I'm not. Too often, I expect you to get the hint and that isn't fair.

9. I need my emergency candies—please don't eat them!

WHAT A LOVED ONE MAY WANT THE PERSON WITH DIABETES TO KNOW

1. I find frequent diabetes problems very frustrating because I care so much.

2. I go crazy when you say, "I'm fine," but you're not.

3. Let's discuss your diabetes emergency plans. I want to know when to help and when not to.

4. I need to know where your emergency supplies are kept.

5. I want to offer help if you can't handle the situation alone. Let's discuss this so we both feel comfortable should the need arise.

Don't let diabetes undermine your loving relationships! Learn as much as you can about this condition, how to avoid developing problems, and how to treat them when they occur. Most situations can be handled calmly and are not emergencies at all. Be open with your needs. If you have diabetes, you need to feel confident that you have the support of others, and they need to know how to help you. Discuss what kinds of help you may need before a situation arises. The wrong help can not only hurt the situation but it can strain your relationship, too. Your friendships are important—don't let diabetes destroy them.

Chapter 7

Testing, Testing, and More Testing!

> My daily blood sugar tests make me so nervous. If I am
> too high or too low, I feel like such a failure. And if my wife
> finds out, it's really awful: "What did you do wrong this
> time?" she asks. I hate it. It's like getting called to the
> principal's office every day.
>
> —Ted

Home blood results are not report cards—you can't pass or
fail. Instead, think of your glucose monitor as a personal
weather channel. If the weatherperson says it's chilly, you grab
a sweater or jacket. If your monitor says your glucose is too
low, you take action to bring it back within your target range.

Don't blame yourself or let anyone blame you for test
results outside of the normal range.

Blood glucose results don't measure your overall diabetes control. That's the role of the A1C test (described in
Chapter 5), which measures your average blood glucose
level for the past two to three months. True, home blood
testing can be time consuming, sometimes painful, and occasionally awkward (when done in public), but the information it provides puts you in control and can relieve you and
your loved ones of worry.

> My dad loves to drive. He takes the car everywhere we
> go. Mom and I never worried until he had a blood sugar
> low and bumped into a tree. He has type 1 diabetes and

always guessed what his blood sugar level was at any given time. We didn't realize that he was not testing his blood sugar. We asked him to stop driving but felt awful about trying to take his independence away. Finally, his diabetes educator convinced him to check his blood glucose throughout the day and treat any lows before getting behind the wheel. Mom and I feel so much better, and Dad's much more confident too.

—Bobby

Ask yourself these basic blood glucose monitoring questions:

1. What is my current glucose level?

2. Is this result out of my target range?

3. If abnormal, why am I at this level?

4. How can I improve this result (if abnormal)?

5. How can I avoid this problem in the future?

Invite your partner to join this discussion and the following exercise. The more you understand about blood glucose monitoring, the greater your comfort level will be.

Before You Test

Are you a gambler? Do you rely on guesses to make treatment decisions? If so, watch out for serious mistakes. Many people are convinced that they can feel their blood sugar level, but research shows that these feelings are often wrong. A glucose monitor provides the most accurate information. No machine is perfect, but the results are more reliable than any guess.

Meters have about a 10–15 percent error rate and may be off by as much as 20 percent if the reading is extremely high or low. But this doesn't render your glucose monitor useless. Use it to identify trends. Are you higher at certain times of the day? Are you lower at others? Share any patterns that you find with your healthcare team. They can help you alter your diabetes care plan, if necessary.

Here are some steps to take to improve your meter's accuracy:

1. Don't use outdated test strips.

2. Store your equipment in a dry, cool location away from temperature extremes.

3. Don't leave the cap off of the test strip container any longer than necessary.

4. Calibrate each new pack of test strips with your machine, as directed by the manufacturer.

5. Check your meter's accuracy periodically with the control solution that comes with the meter. See the instruction booklet for directions.

6. Clean any dust, lint, or blood off your meter.

7. Obtain an adequate blood sample using the tips that follow.

Now, you're almost ready to unlock the mystery of your current blood glucose value. Have your loved one run a blood glucose check too. Your partner should know what it feels like to do this every day and how to interpret the results. Invite him or her to join you as you read through this chapter. Go ahead and prick your finger to get a blood sample. If you have trouble obtaining a drop of blood, try the following tricks:

1. Wash your hands in warm water.

2. Hang your testing hand at your side.

3. Massage that hand from your palm down to your fingertips.

4. Take the sample from the side of your fingertip, not the front pad. It is less painful.

5. Avoid touching the area of the test strip that accepts your blood, as your skin's oils might affect the accuracy of the result.

If your meter allows it, take a blood sample from an area other than your fingertip. Popular alternate sites include the upper arm, thigh, calf, fleshy part of the hand, or forearm. Many individuals who take their blood sample from alternate sites find it less painful than using the fingertip.

Analyze Your Results

Jot down your current blood glucose level. Check this with the suggested target levels listed below, or with your personal target range. All ranges are based on the blood's plasma, which is the watery liquid component of whole blood. If your meter gives whole blood readings your results will be about 15 percent lower than the ones listed here. Check your meter's manual to see if it automatically converts the results.

Pre-breakfast check
Suggested level: 90–130 mg/dl*

*Divide mg/dl by 18 to find the mmol/L value.

If you don't have diabetes: < 110 mg/dl

Pre-meal, pre-snack check
Suggested level: 90–130 mg/dl
If you don't have diabetes: < 110 mg/dl

Post-meal blood test
Suggested target level two hours after the first bite of a meal:
< 180 mg/dl
If you don't have diabetes: < 140 mg/dl

At bedtime
Suggested level: 110–150 mg/dl
If you don't have diabetes: < 120 mg/dl

Note: the symbol < means "less than."

How did you do? Was your result higher or lower than expected or were you within your range? Next, determine what your result means. Timing plays a great role in interpreting how you got to the level you are at right now.

Is it before breakfast?

If you just completed a night of sleep (without raiding the refrigerator), you've been in a fasting state, and yesterday's food has little effect on your result. Your blood glucose level at this time is controlled almost exclusively by your body or diabetes medication. Sugar levels are unpredictable at times, and that can be very frustrating. If your blood sugar is high without any obvious cause, then your result is probably not from anything that you have done. If you just ate a huge piece of chocolate cake with lots of icing, you have a possible explanation.

Your result can be affected by:

1. Your diabetes medication.

2. Physical activity. Exercise can lower blood sugar levels for 24–48 hours or even longer.

3. Your current health. Are you developing a cold, flu, or infection? If so, your results may run higher than normal.

4. Hormonal surges during the night.

5. The setting of your insulin pump, if you wear one.

Before breakfast is a great time to check blood glucose levels because it tells a lot about the status of your diabetes. It also helps you and your healthcare team evaluate the effectiveness of your diabetes plan.

Is it before a meal?

Your pre-meal check can help you spot blood glucose patterns and adjust any medication dose to meet your needs at that moment (especially if you use fast-acting insulin). If your blood sugar levels routinely run low before lunch or dinner, your medication regimen may require adjustment, or a between-meal snack should be added to your day. If levels run high, you might need to reduce the carbohydrate content of your current snack, schedule exercise even earlier in the day, or adjust your medication.

Did you just finish eating?

Everyone's level goes up immediately after eating. Your blood glucose levels will rise because you have just put a new source of energy into your body, namely, food. Your body must digest the food for a while before you can observe its full effect on your blood glucose level. Don't check your blood at this time. Wait until two hours after the first bite of your meal, then check.

Is it two hours after your meal?

Glance at your watch when you take the first bite of your meal. In exactly two hours, check your blood. If your sugar level is above your target range for this time, either your food portions were too large, you had too many carbohydrates, or your medication dose was not adequate for the amount you consumed. If you enjoyed an alcoholic beverage with your meal, it may lower your blood glucose (unless you have a sweet drink such as a piña colada), as will most physical activity.

> I've had type 2 diabetes for over six years. I tried to do whatever my doctor asked, but I never understood why. When my educator introduced post-meal testing to me, everything changed. I didn't know that eating could cause my sugar to climb so high. I cut my portions at lunch, and my post-meal level dropped. Wow! I could actually have control over some of the ups and downs of my diabetes.
>
> —Max

Did you just exercise?

As mentioned above, physical activity can lower blood glucose levels. Expect to have a lower level after a challenging workout, unless you are high prior to starting your activity. If you have type 1 diabetes and your glucose level is poorly controlled, over 300 mg/dl (16.7 mmol/L) at the start of your workout, vigorous activity could cause your blood sugar level to climb even higher. Exercise causes the release of several hormones such as epinephrine (also called adrenalin) that work against insulin. If the body doesn't have enough insulin to counter the effects of these hormones, blood sugar levels will climb. This does not commonly occur in type 2 diabetes because some insulin is usually present. If you go low, use the 15 Rule described in Chapter 6 to normalize your level.

Are you feeling ill?

Check your blood if you feel under the weather. We often blame irritability on an abnormal blood sugar level, but mood swings can be from other causes, too. If you are within your target range, diabetes is not to blame. On the other hand, if your level is climbing, you could be getting sick. Your blood glucose may "know" that you are ill before you do.

Are you having a stressful day?

Studies show that stress can, for some people, occasionally cause blood sugar levels to climb. It can also effect how you take care of your diabetes. When stressed, you may do less exercise, check your blood less frequently, and overeat. Each person is unique, but don't be surprised if your monitoring results are elevated when you are stressed out. Try to reduce the stress in your life.

Last year, I opened my own business. While telling my current bosses that I was leaving the firm to start my own company, I began to sweat and feel sick. They weren't taking it well. I was like a son to them and they took my leaving very personally. I assumed that my feelings were a reaction to the hostile environment in the room, but I checked my blood sugar anyway. I couldn't believe it—I was at a whopping 537 mg/dl! I have type 1 diabetes and an A1C of 5.3 percent. My control is superb; I never go high. I searched for some water or something non-caloric to drink and gave myself some additional insulin. My blood sugar control returned to normal after a day or so.

—John

Are you about to retire for the night?

Were you intimate with your loved one? That form of physical activity will lower your blood sugar level, like any other exercise. Worried about tomorrow? The stress may show up as a higher value on your blood glucose meter if you are aggravated.

If your glucose level is low, eat a light snack to lessen the possibility of going even lower while sleeping. Checking at this time will help you avoid surprise blood sugar lows during the night. A blood glucose level reflects more than just food intake or medication. It warns you about impending illness, responds to a stressful day, or lets you know that all is well.

What can cause a high blood sugar test result?

1. Too much food.

2. Not enough medication or insulin.

3. Inadequate physical activity.

4. Illness, surgery, infections, or any type of injury.

5. A glucose monitor error, outdated test strips, etc.

6. Outdated insulin.

What can cause a low blood sugar test result?

1. Not enough food.

2. Too much medication or insulin.

3. Excessive physical activity.

4. Glucose monitor error.

How to Control Blood Sugar

Now that you know your blood sugar level, what do you do if it is not where it should be? First, know your target range. Your healthcare team can help you determine the range that is right for you, or you can refer to the ranges listed earlier in this chapter. If you have type 1 and use fast-acting insulin or an insulin pump, treat abnormal blood sugar levels as suggested in this chapter or by your diabetes team. If you have type 2 and take pills, it may not be necessary to treat every abnormal blood sugar. Note any abnormal blood glucose trends and discuss them with your healthcare provider, who can help you adjust your diabetes care plan.

If levels are higher than desired before a meal:

1. Eat less than your normal amount of food.

2. Delay your meal.

3. Spread out your upcoming meal and save the fruit for later.

4. Exercise lightly; take a walk after your meal.

5. Increase the time between your meal and insulin dose.

If levels are higher than desired after a meal:

1. Take additional medication or insulin as directed by your healthcare team.

2. Participate in a light activity like walking.

3. Delay your upcoming snack.

4. Drink plenty of water.

If you are low at any time, use the 15 Rule to return your blood glucose levels to normal (see Chapter 6) and try to avoid the cause of the problem in the future.

Check your blood at the same time of day for several days to see if a pattern appears. If your abnormal blood sugar level happens repeatedly, adjust your care plan. Meet with your healthcare team to discuss the options for change. You may need to alter your meal plan, physical activity schedule and intensity, or medication.

How Do You Feel about Testing?

Find a healthy balance between the number of blood checks you believe you should take and the number that fit comfortably into your life. Diabetes doesn't go away, so achieving good control should blend into your life and not become an impossible burden.

Not everyone tests frequently, and not everyone needs to. Individuals who control their diabetes with exercise and diet alone can do quite well with fewer checks, perhaps once a day or a few times a week. Those who take insulin injections or use an insulin pump, may require multiple daily glucose checks to match their insulin to their individual needs. Speak with your healthcare provider to determine the amount of testing that is right for you.

Now, take an honest look at how you feel about daily blood glucose testing. What fits into your personal comfort zone? Remember, tasks that help achieve good control should not stress you or the relationships that you have with the ones you love.

If you have diabetes, jot down your answers to the following questions:

1. How many times a day do I need to check my blood sugar?

2. How do I use the results?

3. What testing times do I find difficult and why?

4. What can my partner do to help make testing easier (examples: staying nearby to offer emotional support, going to the pharmacy for supplies, writing results in a booklet)?

If you love someone with diabetes, jot down your answers to these questions:

1. How often should my partner check his or her blood sugar?

2. Do I feel confident that my partner knows what to do with the results?

3. At what times does my partner find it difficult to check his or her blood sugar?

4. What can I do to make it easier for my partner to test?

5. I'd like to help my partner with his or her blood sugar checking. When we get together with friends, I could help make the environment more supportive by statements like:

> "While (s)he is testing, why don't we all decide to order?"

> "Oh, (s)he will be done soon. Don't worry. It's no big deal."

> "When you're done checking your blood, tell us what you want to order."

Can you think of other ways of being supportive and helpful?

Share your answers. Does your partner know you as well as you thought? Did you learn anything new about each other?

Technological advances make it easier to do tasks that used to be quite intrusive. Blood glucose monitoring used to be a messy and lengthy event. Today's meters require smaller samples of blood than ever before, provide results in as little time as five seconds, and some contain their own test strips that magically appear with a push of a button.

WHAT A PERSON WITH DIABETES MAY WANT HIS OR HER FRIENDS TO KNOW

1. Testing is not fun.

2. Sometimes I don't want anyone—including me—to see the results.

3. Please don't rush me while I am trying to test and don't discourage me from testing if you are in a hurry. My blood checks are important and help me stay healthy.

4. If you are uncomfortable with the sight of blood, look away. I don't want to leave the table each time I check. I want to enjoy the conversation with my friends.

WHAT A LOVED ONE MAY WANT THE PERSON WITH DIABETES TO KNOW

1. I wish you'd share your results with me. I want to help.

2. I don't always understand your need for repetitive blood checks. Please tell me how they improve your diabetes control.

3. I may become impatient if your daily tasks make me late for appointments. Please schedule these activities so I can leave on time.

4. I may become uncomfortable around blood. Please be as discreet as possible.

5. I'd like to help others be more comfortable when you are checking your blood.

6. Please tell me how I can help.

Daily diabetes tasks can be overwhelming to everyone in your life. Work with your healthcare provider to choose the blood-monitoring times that best fit into your lifestyle and give you and your healthcare team the most valuable information. Don't forget to communicate their rationale with the ones who love you. They are sure to be comforted by your understanding and command of these challenging situations.

Don't let blood sugar checks cause arguments between you and your loved ones. If tests indicate that you are out of your target range, it doesn't mean that you've "been bad." Your test result is just information, not a statement about your worth as a human being. Diabetes can be a frustrating condition. Sometimes you do all the right things—eat well, exercise, and take the correct amount of medication—but your diabetes remains difficult to control.

Supporting your loved one who has diabetes, as he or she takes these important checks, can bring great rewards: good health, fewer possible complications, and reduced worry. Not a bad investment.

Chapter 8

Does the Checkout Lady Need to Know?

You don't have to tell everyone you meet that you or someone close to you has diabetes. It is very personal information. As the incidence of diabetes continues to grow, people are becoming more comfortable and open with the topic. But it is still totally up to the person with diabetes to decide how and when to share the news.

Whom Should You Tell?

It is up to you to choose who needs to know. When deciding, remember that most people want the best for you and want to help you with potential problems that arise in your life. If you wish to share your news, here are some folks who might be worth telling:

a. People who can assist you with your diabetes care.

b. Anyone who can provide emotional support.

c. Those who need to know your medical condition, such as an exercise instructor, scuba diving teacher, and other health professionals.

d. An employer—especially if you need to ask for special schedules, break times, or time off for medical appointments.

e. Someone with whom you share an intimate relationship.

f. Roommates.

g. Workout buddies, who may see you go low and can offer help.

At the end of a long hike in Hawaii, Bill and Chris were about one mile from their destination. Suddenly, Chris' behavior began to change. He walked slower and slower, studying each step as he took it. Luckily, Bill knew that Chris had type 1 diabetes and suspected that his blood sugar levels were dropping. He remembered that Chris had tossed some peanut M&Ms into his bag in case of a hypoglycemic emergency but was stubborn and unlikely to admit that one was really taking place. Chris' mood worsened with every step. Bill knew that any mention of a possible low would definitely start a fight. So Bill decided to be a bit cagey about it:

Bill: Hey Chris, where are those peanut M&Ms? It would be nice to open them up right now.

Chris: Bill! You know that those are for when I go low. Don't touch them!

Chris got progressively worse. He became even more unsteady, so Bill pushed even harder for the candy.

Bill: Chris, I'd love to have some candy. You obviously don't need any and I'm really hungry.

Chris: Who are you to tell me whether or not I need them? You know, now that I think about it, I might be getting low. I think I will have a few.

Chris checked his blood sugar. It was 40 mg/dl.

Who Does Not Need to Know?

a. Anyone who will nag you.

b. A person who will offer tempting foods that you prefer to avoid.

c. Anyone who will make fun of any lifestyle changes that you make.

d. Someone who might gossip about you.

e. A person who would be a source of constant criticism.

f. Someone who just won't understand.

g. A person you barely know or don't know at all.

h. Someone with whom you feel uncomfortable discussing personal matters.

Mark is 45, has had type 2 diabetes for about two years, and still hasn't told his parents.

> I'm sure they would drive me crazy. They always blow things out of proportion and lose sleep over every worry. They will research everything that they can find on it and bore me with endless stories of acquaintances that have lost legs to diabetes and other horror stories. Just what I need! Worst of all, they will spread the news to all of their friends.

If you are the spouse or partner of a person with diabetes, you have the option to share or not to share the news, but with one important caveat: respect your loved one's request to keep the news away from certain individuals. Don't go behind his or her back and share it anyway. Imagine the damage if someone you told spots your partner and accidentally mentions the condition. It could damage the trust that the two of you have built, cause your partner to withhold future information, create a rift that may not heal quickly, or even encourage your loved one to confide in someone else instead of you. If your loved one doesn't want some people to know, don't tell them!

How to Discuss Diabetes

How you tell the news to others is as important as to whom you tell it. If you aren't careful, all could go wrong. Jordon was unable to communicate details about his diabetes to Gayle in an appealing way and the end result was disastrous:

> Jordon was a nervous wreck, but not from his diabetes, which he had lived with for 13 years. Tonight was supposed to be the night. He kept reaching into his pocket every few seconds to make certain that the engagement ring was still there. He had been planning this moment for weeks and wanted everything to be perfect. He knew Gayle was the woman for him from the first minute that he met her 10 months ago, and it was now time to move forward.
>
> Sadly, the night did not go as planned. At the restaurant, when he opened the velvet box containing the engagement ring and popped the question, Gayle just sat there. Finally she said, "Jordon, I've been thinking about this for a long time. I love you, but I can't handle your diabetes. All I know about it is that you have it and curse it out every chance you get. I've never heard you say anything positive about it at all. If it is as bad as you say it is, I don't want to live with it, either. I'm sorry. I won't marry you."

Those who hear your story will gauge their response based on your attitude. If you are fearful about having diabetes, the people you tell might become scared also. If you are calm, relaxed and confident, they will feel that way too. You set the tone. Unfortunately, Jordon neglected to communicate to Gayle that it was possible to live a fulfilling and successful life with diabetes. His negative feelings turned her off.

A diabetes educator retells this story about a patient who was diagnosed with diabetes a year earlier but had not shared the news with her family:

> Several of my patient's relatives had recently died from diabetes. To help deal with their loss, she took her 13-year-old son to a program for relatives of people with diabetes. Before entering the room, she took him aside and told him that she too had diabetes. Fortunately, the class presented diabetes in a very positive light. They said that it did not have to be a terrible burden or death sentence for anyone. They both left feeling upbeat and my patient decided to inform the rest of the family about her diabetes that weekend at a family barbecue. The news was presented in a relaxing environment and everyone took it well.

Your Spouse or Partner

Your partner or spouse will probably be your closest supporter on this new journey. You probably heard the news together or shared the diagnosis immediately after receiving it. In that initial state of shock, the information you related may have just poured out of you with all of your fears, worries, anger, and disappointment, which is appropriate since your partner is probably your most intimate confidant. You need to be open and honest with that person, and any way you break the news is probably just fine. Once you both know the diagnosis, however, race quickly to the positives:

a. Diabetes does not have to shorten your life.

b. You do not have to develop complications.

c. Your children are not doomed to develop diabetes.

d. You can absolutely, positively still fulfill all of your dreams and goals.

e. Having diabetes can enhance the quality of your life by encouraging you to eat in a healthier manner, exercise regularly, and have regular check-ups.

f. Diabetes can improve the lives of your entire family, as you all take on a healthier lifestyle.

Close Relatives and Friends

Good buddies and close family members who understand diabetes can play a terrific role in your support system. They help you recognize problems, assist with diabetes care, offer emotional support, and can call for emergency assistance if needed. Practice what to say and, above all, know your facts so you respond effectively to the many myths about diabetes.

> Patrick: Hey, Kevin, I just learned that I have diabetes. I don't know everything about it yet, but I do know that if I take care of it, which I will, it shouldn't cause me any serious problems.

> Kevin: Wow. What about amputations? My aunt lost her leg to diabetes. Don't you have to eat differently? Are you going to need insulin shots?

> Patrick: They now know so much more about how to prevent complications. I have a great doctor and will go to classes to learn exactly what I need to do.

> Kevin: Is there anything that I can do to help?

> Patrick: I don't know yet, but if I need anything I will definitely ask. Thanks for offering.

If you wish, invite your friend to join you at your diabetes classes. Or, share copies of materials that you receive and discuss them together. Remember, the attitude that you bring sets the tone.

Dating

Diabetes is hardly a romantic topic, but it is an important one to share when searching for a life partner. Perhaps Jordon and Gayle would be on their way down the aisle today had he been able to talk about his diabetes in a more relaxed and confident manner. Here are some successful ways in which different individuals have introduced their diabetes to their dates:

JILL AND KYLE

It was our first date and we were both a bit nervous. We sat down in the restaurant and Kyle placed a white plastic toothbrush holder on the table. My first thought was, "Wow, this guy cares a lot about oral hygiene!" When I asked about the holder, he nonchalantly answered that it contained his insulin and then went back to reading the menu.

Before meeting Kyle, if someone had asked me to date a person with diabetes, I probably would have said no—it is a serious medical condition that I knew nothing about. But seeing how comfortable he was, assured me that it was no problem.

Kyle didn't write "I Have Diabetes" across his forehead but conveyed the information in a relaxed, comfortable way. Jill was impressed with his confident attitude, which quickly put her at ease. They were married less than a year later.

JON

Jon prefers to jump right in. He has had type 1 diabetes since the age of 16. He truly believes that it is no big deal and, like Kyle, prefers to let his behavior do the talking. He routinely pulls out his glucose meter and tests his blood right in front of his dates, which always spurs a lively discussion. Some women are comfortable, others less so. The conversation that follows is always enlightening and gives Jon a chance to help another person understand the real facts about diabetes.

CYNDEE

Cyndee is less subtle. She beams a generous smile and says, "I believe in honesty, so I want to share something about myself with you. I have type 1 diabetes and have had it for many years. Do you know anyone else with type 1 diabetes?" This comment usually starts a great discussion. Cyndee listens for misunderstandings and then decides how to proceed. Most of her encounters have led to meaningful exchanges, memorable relationships, and, yes, even a few rejections.

Not everyone is comfortable with the topic of diabetes as shown by the following story:

TINA AND GREG

Tina spent months trying to get Greg's attention. When he finally asked her out, she was sure that he was "the one." On their date, she told him about her diabetes and he suddenly became very quiet and then lost interest in their conversation. "I can't pinpoint exactly what happened, but I knew from his reaction that he wasn't going to ask me out again. I guess I should thank my diabetes for exposing his lack of sensitivity and letting me know that he wasn't for me.

Diabetes and Your Children

Kids need to know about your diabetes, especially if they live with you. They will observe you doing diabetes care tasks, exercising, eating differently, and working to meet your diabetes goals. They will pick up on your fears and could become fearful, too. They need information and guidance, as their lives may also be affected.

A diabetes-friendly home contains healthy food and encourages everyone to participate in regular physical activity, which promotes good health. If your children are overweight, inactive, and used to eating generous amounts of junk food, their lives may change dramatically, much to their chagrin. They need to understand what is happening so they can support these household changes and enjoy future good health. Here are a few helpful strategies to help you break the news to your little ones.

Come Prepared

Review the basics of diabetes before bringing up the topic. Come to this discussion prepared so you can answer the questions that your children ask.

Show How You Haven't Changed

You are the same person you have always been; diabetes doesn't make you different. With good care, you are still likely to live a long and healthy life. Diabetes may alter your schedule a bit, but it doesn't have to affect the activities that you and your kids do together. You can still share many new and exciting adventures.

Get Your Kids Involved

Involve the children in your diabetes care but don't overdo it. Invite them to assist you when you inspect your feet. Have them help you decide what to eat. Your relaxed demeanor sends the message that all is well. Be careful not to over-involve your children. They don't have to learn about every possible complication or physical symptom. The goal is to include them and enlist their support, not scare them.

Jeanette was diagnosed with gestational diabetes early in her third pregnancy. She was asked to follow a strict meal program and check her blood four times each day. Instead of checking in private, she enlisted her daughters, Carol and Tanya, ages 3 and 6, respectively, to assist her. "Carol's job was to bring me my glucose meter and Talia wrote down the results in a notebook. Both sang along whenever the meter went "Beep" and cheered when my blood sugar was where it was supposed to be. If my result wasn't good, they told me that I would do better next time!"

Kathy, on the other hand, invited her 9-year-old daughter, Jill, to become a bit too involved in Kathy's diabetes world. She thought it would be educational to have Jill assist with her insulin injections. When some bleeding appeared at the injection site, Jill became scared and refused to help with any future diabetes tasks.

Allow Children to Share the News

Give your children the option to tell a few of their friends. Remind them that there is no need to be embarrassed because diabetes isn't a shameful secret. Sharing this information with a best friend or two can be very helpful for them.

Be Positive and Honest

Be open and upbeat. Explain how having diabetes reminds you to take care of yourself and stay healthy. It is no big deal as long as you take care of yourself, which you plan to do. Just as your children's friends take medicine to control their allergies or asthma, you will take what you need to control your diabetes. Wonderful treatments are available and you have a healthcare team that oversees your care.

Be honest about the changes that will be happening in the house:

a. Explain why the entire family's eating habits may have to change but that eating well and staying active will help them be healthy, strong, and full of energy.

b. Enlist the children's help in a whirlwind effort to get unhealthy foods out of the house. Have them place unopened food in bags for donation to a local food bank. Not only will they become more familiar with healthier food choices but they will learn about giving to others.

c. Have them shop with you and learn to read food labels.

d. Invite the kids to help plan well-balanced meals and snacks and participate in food preparation.

e. Participate in physical activities together—do an exercise video, bike, play tennis, go for a swim, rollerblade, hike, etc.

f. Most of all, teach your children to respect and support everyone's effort to live a healthier life.

Diabetes and Your Workplace

Not everyone in the office needs to know that you have diabetes, but a few knowledgeable coworkers can make a difference. They can help make sure that office celebrations include food choices that you can enjoy, and give you a "heads up" if you display any low blood-sugar symptom, like extreme fatigue and irritability. Let your chosen workmates know where you keep your emergency phone numbers, your glucagon kit (with instructions), and low blood-sugar snack foods. Inform all that these items are exclusively for your use.

Your Boss

Through the grapevine, Marty learned that rumors had been spreading about his increased absences and inability to concentrate on projects assigned to him. He went to his doctor to examine his recent weight loss and discovered that he had type 2 diabetes. With medication, he soon began to feel himself again. To stop the rumors from growing, he felt it important to disclose his diabetes to his boss.

> It was a tough conversation, one that I didn't want to have. I feel that personal business should stay personal. I'm not close with my boss but believed it important for him to know the truth about my health. He was very understanding and shared some of his medical history with me, too. With his help, the rumors lost their steam and went away.

It is not always necessary to tell your boss that you have diabetes, but sometimes it must be done. In a perfect world, this discussion would go well and your boss would become an enthusiastic advocate for your medical needs. But what if it doesn't go well? Many laws protect your rights in the workplace, but most anti-discrimination laws only offer protection if your employer is aware of your condition.

Your Rights

The following is a general summary of some of the rights that a person with diabetes has. We are not lawyers, but feel it is worthwhile that you know there are important laws on your side. For additional information, contact the American Diabetes Association (ADA). It has a superb advocacy section on its website, www.diabetes.org. You can also contact them by calling 1-800-DIABETES to find out about the rights you have in your particular state.

Anti-discrimination laws prohibit an employer from discriminating against a person with diabetes or any disability in the following areas:

a. hiring

b. firing

c. discipline

d. pay

e. promotion

f. job training

g. fringe benefits

Employers are required to make "reasonable accommodation" if an employee with a disability requests it but don't have to comply with a request that creates "undue hardship" because of its difficulty to implement or expense. But certain adjustments are easy and should be done to help you handle diabetes in your workplace:

a. Permitting you to eat while working.

b. Allowing for frequent breaks to check blood glucose levels, take a snack, or visit the bathroom.

c. Permission to keep diabetes supplies and snacks handy.

d. Freedom to work a modified schedule or a standard shift instead of a split or swing shift that would cause timing challenges with your care.

Anti-Discrimination Laws

These laws prohibit discrimination in the workplace when you have a disability like diabetes. We don't think of diabetes as a disability, but the law does. Here are two important federal laws:

1. The Americans with Disabilities Act applies to private employers, labor unions, state and local government, and agencies with 15 or more employees.

2. The Rehabilitation Act of 1973 covers employees who work for the executive branch of the federal government or an employer who receives federal funds.

Each state also has its own set of anti-discrimination laws. Contact the ADA at 1-800-DIABETES and ask to speak with the ADA contact for your state to find out about your rights under both state and federal laws.

The Family and Medical Leave Act (FMLA)

Most government and private employers with more than 50 employees must provide up to 12 weeks of job-protected but unpaid leave each year for a serious health condition of either an employee or a member of his or her family. This time off does not have to be used all at one time and can be apportioned to handle short-term problems related to blood sugar levels or doctor's appointments.

How to Take Action

If you believe that you or a loved one is being discriminated against at work because of diabetes, try the following:

a. Contact the ADA, your union, or an attorney.

b. Keep copies of all documents that pertain to your claim, such as a memo from your boss.

c. Get copies of other general documents that may be important, such as personnel policy statements.

d. Keep a journal and write down everything that happens to you at work. Include specific names and dates.

Problems often occur because a boss is ignorant about diabetes and your rights. Many difficulties can be worked out by sharing information about your condition and medical needs. Bring articles that support your request. Manufacturers of particular items, such as insulin pumps, can supply you with research articles on the value of their products.

Submit any request you make of your employer in writing, and include information on how it will enhance your diabetes management. Mention that these products or actions will reduce your likelihood of complications, and your improved care will result in better productivity and a financial savings for the company.

If your employer is not familiar with anti-discrimination laws, you can provide this information as well. If problems continue, it may be necessary to file a discrimination charge against your employer. The ADA should be able to help you contact the right individuals to proceed.

Recruiting Diabetes Advocates

If you are up to it, help spread the word about diabetes.

> Entertainer Barry Gibb of the Bee Gees and his wife, Linda, moved to the Miami area over 20 years ago. There, they befriended a neighbor whose son had diabetes. They talked about a variety of diabetes issues. Barry's grandmother also had the disease, so Barry and Linda's interest quickly blossomed into generous and enthusiastic support. Today, they are the International Chairs of the University of Miami's Diabetes Research Institute, a recognized world leader in cure-focused research and pioneer in islet cell transplants. The Gibbs now contribute to the research center and Barry frequently performs at the DRI's annual fundraiser.

Research and education need the support of generous donors and volunteers. Invite friends and family members to diabetes walk-a-thons and other educational and charitable events. If you prefer to be more private about this, tell only a few chosen coworkers and good friends.

WHAT A PERSON WITH DIABETES MAY WANT HIS OR HER FRIENDS TO KNOW

1. I don't want to tell everyone about my diabetes. Sometimes it is more comfortable to tell just a few so I don't have to deal with innumerable questions and comments.

2. You do not decide who I tell. It is my prerogative, not yours.

3. I may surprise you by choosing to tell certain individuals about my diabetes. Sometimes I'm in the mood to share this with others, sometimes not.

WHAT A LOVED ONE MAY WANT THE PERSON WITH DIABETES TO KNOW

1. It may be tough at times, but I will do my best to respect your need to stay silent about your condition. I may need to talk to someone about it, too, so let's discuss whom I can tell.

2. I want to learn as much about diabetes as possible. Mutual friends might ask me questions about it.

Discussing diabetes with others can be a challenge, but it doesn't have to be. People come to this topic with many misconceptions and concerns. Learn all you can about diabetes. Practice what you plan to say and how you would like to present it. Remember, through your words and actions, you set the tone that cues others how to respond. If you are relaxed, most of those around you will be as well.

Diabetes doesn't have to be a horrible secret. Telling others can bring comfort and support to all of you.

Chapter 9

Mind Your P's and Q's

Do you practice proper diabetes etiquette? Did you even know it existed? Apparently, some people do know—and get quite irate when it is ignored:

> Dear Ann Landers:
> I have a relative who has diabetes and must take insulin shots after* every meal. He makes quite a production of it, tests his sugar, prepares the injection, and injects himself at the table. This procedure is done in the homes of family members and friends and in restaurants. The sight of blood and injections ruins the enjoyment of the meal for those with queasy stomachs.
> This person is extremely sensitive, and his feelings would be crushed if he knew he was offending people. Your response in the paper would help make others who are afflicted with diabetes aware of how this sort of thing affects some of us.
> —Mrs. Anonymous
> *Insulin is usually taken before meals.

Ann Landers' response:

> Dear Mrs. Anon:
> Your point is well taken. A person who would inject himself or herself at the dinner table in the presence of others exhibits gross insensitivity and very poor manners.

Ms. Landers had very strong ideas about diabetes etiquette, but was she right? We don't think so. A person who injects in public does not show "gross insensitivity and very poor manners"; however, there are right and wrong ways to handle your diabetes when others are around.

What Exactly Is Diabetes Etiquette?

Diabetes etiquette isn't about table settings, thank-you notes, or keeping elbows off the table. It's about behavior that helps everyone become comfortable with diabetes and does not embarrass the person who has it.

Here are some examples:

If you have diabetes:

1. Make your needs known in a polite yet effective way.

2. Be considerate of others when performing diabetes tasks in public, such as insulin injections and blood glucose checks.

3. Be considerate of restaurant staff and those dining with you when you make special foods requests.

4. Offer hosts information about your food needs in advance to avoid any awkward entertaining moments. Most people appreciate this helpful advice; if they prepare something you prefer not to eat, it could be uncomfortable for all of you.

If you care about someone with diabetes:

1. Try to make it easier for your loved one. Don't nag.

2. If you don't know or understand something about diabetes, ask.

3. Treat your loved one like any other person. Don't make a big deal about special requirements.

4. Try to be more understanding than Ann Landers!

Going Public

It can be awkward and uncomfortable for you or for others when you inject insulin in public. Do you do it at meetings or in restaurants? It can be cumbersome to prepare a syringe, and the sight of it may send an observer's stomach into a tailspin. You could leave the table and the conversation you are having, but that option isn't fair. You shouldn't have to hide your diabetes or be punished for it.

You are at an elegant restaurant with relatives and your food has just arrived. You know how much fast-acting insulin you need and prepare to inject it. Your cousin sees what you are doing and asks you to please leave the table. What should you do? What would you say? See if you agree on how to handle this situation.

Here's our response: The timing of insulin injections is important. One should not delay an injection just to make a relative happy. No one expects individuals to seek a private spot to take aspirin or use an asthma inhaler. Your insulin needs should be respected as well.

But a restaurant is not the place to begin a heated discussion about diabetes. Nevertheless, leaving the table shouldn't be necessary. Try saying, "This will just take a second." Then turn away and inject into an inconspicuous spot on your leg or in your abdomen that is hidden by the table. When the time feels right, talk about diabetes if you wish.

Here are some additional ways to keep your injections private and out of the public eye:

Choose Your Injection Site Well

Some locations on the body are better in public than others; the thigh is more hidden than the buttocks or arm, for example. Steve, one of our authors, has his favorite injection spot right below the knee, on the inside of his leg. Here's how to do it:

1. Cross your right leg over your left.

2. Lift your pant leg and locate the fatty area found on the left side of your right leg, just below the knee.

3. Inject.

Use an Insulin Pen

Specially made pen-sized insulin devices are used by 90–95 percent of insulin-treated patients in Europe, Scandinavia, and Asia. The pens contain a reservoir of insulin and a small, replaceable needle. To use, attach a new needle to the end, dial up the desired amount, and press the button. The injection is automatic and pain is minimized because the needle is not pushed through the thick rubber top of an insulin bottle, so it stays sharp. It is much less painful than pricking a finger for blood sugar checks.

Few American patients use pens, which is unfortunate because they are so convenient to use: They're small and resemble pens, they hide insulin well, and they can give a quick and discreet injection. The plastic or metal covers also protect the insulin from heat and light, preventing it from losing potency over time.

Special Requests of Friends and Family

How about special food requests at home and with other family members? Sometimes it is much easier to ask questions of a waiter you won't see again. Family members tend to take these things very personally.

> I spend Thanksgiving at my aunt's every year. She always cooks up a storm and goes out of her way to make diabetes-friendly foods for me. That alone would be wonderful, but the story doesn't end there. She then takes all of these luscious foods and puts them on a separate table, decorated especially for me. When I enter her home, she always greets me by saying, "Bob, it is so great to see you! Your special buffet table is over here." I love my aunt and appreciate all the trouble she goes to, but I hate being singled out and treated differently.
>
> —Bob

Bob hasn't figured out how to resolve this problem yet. If he continues to keep his feelings to himself, the relationship that he has with his aunt may disintegrate altogether without her ever knowing why. What advice can you offer him? How should he tell her about his needs?

We suggest a simple solution: Bob should offer to come a few hours early and help set up. When his aunt brings up the topic of his special foods, he can nonchalantly answer that he can enjoy all of the foods that she serves, so there is no need to set up a special table for him. If she asks why this is so, he can use her question as a way to begin a discussion of the new diabetes meal planning philosophies—how he can eat anything as long as he watches his portions, how sugar is now permitted on a diabetic meal plan, and that the foods on his meal plan are healthy for everyone. Finally, he should be honest with her. He should thank her for trying so hard to meet his needs but let her know that having his own table embarrasses him a bit, even though he realizes that she is doing it out of love.

How do you politely make your food needs known to others?

> I'm having a housewarming party for my niece who has diabetes. This is her first home and I want to make something really special for her. I heard that she might not be able to eat cake, which I typically prepare for this kind of an event. I have absolutely no idea what to serve. Can I make my cake? Would it be rude if I did? Maybe it would hurt her feelings. Do I have to buy special foods for her? Can we have cocktails? I'm stumped.
>
> —Sarah

What would you suggest and how would you say it? Here's our suggestion:

Desserts are not off limits for those with diabetes, but a varied menu will make everyone comfortable. Add fruit and vegetable platters to the menu, along with simple desserts like cookies. Our real concern is Sarah's discomfort. She feels lost not knowing what to serve and doesn't seem to know where to head for information.

If friends throw a party for you or host an event that you plan to attend, make their life easier with a phone call. Call and ask about the menu. Give them a chance to ask about your needs, and let them know that you would like to make your own food choices from the things offered at the party. Anticipate their discomfort and head it off at the pass. People do want to do the right thing. Help them.

People are more health conscious these days, but that doesn't always carry over to entertaining. Some believe that holidays and celebrations are great excuses to fall off the health wagon. Hosts may fill their buffet tables with fried and high-calorie everything and then spend the balance of the evening discussing the latest weight-loss craze.

If you arrive expecting to enjoy fresh vegetables and healthy entrees, you might be disappointed, so prepare for the worst. Carry snacks or eat in advance. If a friend leaves you out of meal planning decisions for an event, it can cause an uncomfortable evening. Don't let it. Use the situation as an opportunity to educate.

Discourage Snack Sneakers

Myron is tired of the constant food fights that go on in his house. His diet soda disappears and his favorite sugar-free fudge pops evaporate magically into thin air. His family eats what he buys and leaves none for him. What should he do? What should he say? Here is our suggestion:

Myron should discuss his feelings with his family and have his items set aside and labeled for his personal diabetes use. Since everyone loves Myron's food so much, he could buy additional supplies for the rest of the family. Myron's wife might tell him that the family thinks he is too possessive of the snack foods and beverages. Don't let the anger grow. Talk it out and avoid the war.

Set a time to convey the feelings of everyone in the household. Acknowledge that everyone appreciates his needs, but with limited pantry space, all must do a better job of sharing. One suggestion might be to label and set aside some items for Myron and leave the rest for all who want it. Ask Myron what he suggests. Discuss the options that he comes up with, and decide which options to try. What is healthy for him is healthy for the rest of the family! Remember to keep a cool head and be as dispassionate as possible.

How Can You Make Your Needs Known Without a Fuss?

You don't have to tell everyone the details of your life, but a few friends and relatives can be a great help. They can lobby for reasonably timed lunch breaks and flexible schedules at work. They can ask that diabetes-friendly food be available at family gatherings. They can assist you in an emergency and help you with diabetes care tasks. A request is not the same as a demand, but sometimes loved ones do feel put upon by the person with diabetes.

> I can't take it. I feel like I have no life anymore. George calls my name over and over to ask for a whole list of things. "Bring me my glucose monitor." "I feel low, bring me some juice." "Take my blood, I hate doing it." "Check my feet." Really! He was always such a strong man, but after having type 2 diabetes for over 3 years, he has turned into a little child. Sometimes, when I hear my name, I absolutely cringe. I know that these things are important and I am proud that I am there for him. But some days, I'm telling you, I just can't stand it. I wish he would do these things for himself. After all, he is a grown man!
>
> —Dolores

How do you ask for help? Do you request or demand it? Are you pleased when help finally arrives or annoyed that it took too long? How do you think that diabetes care requests should be worded? Here is our suggestion:

Be very specific when you make a request. Don't expect your loved one to read your mind or know exactly how to do a particular task. Thank those who help you. They need to understand your situation, but consideration by both of you goes a long way.

Clean Up Your Act

Are you considerate with your diabetes materials at home? If you leave your tools or garbage around, you might be setting yourself up for a future battle. Our authors have their own story:

> The three of us had our first meeting for this book in a hotel lounge at a San Francisco hotel. An acquaintance stopped in to say hello. In the middle of the conversation, he pulled out his blood glucose monitor and proceeded to sample his blood and run a glucose check. Being healthcare professionals, we totally understand the need to check in public. What

we didn't understand was the pile of testing "garbage" that he left on our table when he exited the room: his used test strip, lancet, and blood-stained cotton ball.

—Janis, Bill, and Steve

Do your items on the nightstand, kitchen counter, and bathroom sink bother your family? Open and honest communication, with a generous dose of de-cluttering, should help defuse this potentially explosive situation. Here are some suggestions:

- Keep out the diabetes supplies that you use routinely. Store the rest out of sight in closets and cabinets and drawers.

- Keep the materials that you use each day in decorative containers.

- Throw used lancets and other blood-tinged items into a specially made container immediately after using.

- Clean up your mess! Otherwise you will drive friends and family crazy.

Nothing drives my wife crazier then finding my used strips on the floor of my car, in my coat pocket, etc. I have now been trained to dispose of them properly.

—Steven

If you are the loved one who lives with a household of diabetes paraphernalia, try the following:

- Share how you feel about having diabetes messes around. Don't accuse, just highlight how a clean and tidy environment is good for both of you and more hygienic, too.

- Purchase attractive storage containers for diabetes materials.

- Clear away other, non-diabetes items like books and magazines. It is difficult to see the size of a mess if it is hidden by other things.

- Have patience. New behaviors take time.

- Praise positive changes.

Watch Your Language

There are also etiquette rules for those who do not have diabetes:

1. It is not your place to remind a loved one with diabetes how to eat properly.

2. If your partner with diabetes is angry, don't automatically blame it on his or her condition.

3. Do not treat anyone who is newly diagnosed with diabetes like they have suddenly become fragile or stupid. Neither is true.

4. Don't blame the person with diabetes for his or her blood sugar highs or lows. They can happen for a variety of reasons that cannot be controlled.

WHAT A PERSON WITH DIABETES MAY WANT HIS OR HER FRIENDS TO KNOW

1. I want you to know all about diabetes etiquette without my having to tell you.

2. Please ask me if you don't know what I should or shouldn't eat or what kinds of needs I have.

3. I like to be treated like everyone else.

4. I will do my best to practice my diabetes care in a way that is comfortable for everyone.

WHAT A LOVED ONE MAY WANT THE PERSON WITH DIABETES TO KNOW

1. I may ask you about your diabetes needs, especially if we are serving food at an event.

2. Please let me know if I can do something to make diabetes easier for you.

3. If I offend you, it is unintentional. Please let me know.

4. I like to feel appreciated when I offer to help.

Diabetes etiquette is nothing more than being considerate and tolerant of others who are different. Whether you have diabetes or not, at some point you will probably be in a situation where you won't know the polite or proper thing to do. The solution? Start a conversation; those around you will clue you in on the correct way to act. Few people understand the needs of those who live with diabetes every day, but that is the challenge: to let people know (in a gracious way) that diabetes fits in anywhere and should be allowed everywhere.

Chapter 10

Sex and Other Fun Stuff

> After fifteen years of marriage, they finally achieved sexual compatibility. They both had a headache.
>
> —From *Kosher Sex* by Shmeuli Boteach
> (Doubleday, 1999)

No one's sex life is perfect. Well, at least no one we know. If you have problems with your sex life, you are not alone. Many people, with and without diabetes, have occasional sexual problems, but diabetes makes them more likely to occur.

> When I was diagnosed with type 2 a few months ago, I ignored the whole thing. As long as I didn't take shots, I figured it wasn't serious. Then I started having trouble in the bedroom, if you know what I mean. That did it for me. I didn't walk, I ran to make an appointment with my doctor. He was booked up, so I met with a diabetes educator the next day. Fortunately, no other patients were waiting, so he had time to discuss it with me and presented many excellent treatment options.
>
> —Ivan

You can avoid developing most diabetes-related sexual problems by maintaining good diabetes control, as discussed in detail in previous chapters. If you are already running into problems affecting erection, lubrication, and libido, don't despair. Excellent treatments are available.

Erection Difficulties

Occasional erection problems happen to most men. If you can't maintain an erection long enough to have successful intercourse in over half of your attempts, you have "erectile dysfunction" or "ED." It was formerly called impotence, which is an inaccurate and unfair term. Impotence implies that something is wrong with your masculinity, that you are a weak person and are less of a man because you can't perform sexually. Not true. ED is the most common sexual side effect of diabetes; it occurs in many men and becomes more likely as one gets older.

An erection begins when a man becomes sexually aroused from a touch, a thought, something seen, or even something heard. Nerves from the brain and skin send messages to the penis, which allows blood to enter but not exit. Like a water balloon, the penis will grow in size and stiffen. It is difficult to perform sexually if an adequate amount of blood cannot reach and stay in the penis. This happens if circulation problems exist or if the body's nerve messages are blocked.

> Dave and Laura planned the perfect evening, but everything had gone wrong again. The kids were at their grandparents', a candlelight dinner was set, and soothing music was drifting in softly. Once again, Dave, who has had type 1 diabetes for over 20 years, had been unable to maintain an adequate erection for longer than a few minutes. It didn't happen every time but was becoming too frequent. He couldn't bring himself to speak to anyone about this, not even Laura. They both began to worry.

Do you have ED? Take the following quiz, based on the Sexual Health Inventory for Men (SHIM) quiz from the Viagra.com website:

A. *How do you rate your confidence that you can achieve and keep an erection?*

1. Very low

2. Low

3. Moderate

4. High

5. Very high

B. *When you have erections with sexual stimulation, how often are your erections hard enough for penetration (entering your partner)?*

0. No sexual activity

1. Almost never or never

2. A few times (much less than half the time)

3. Sometimes (about half the time)

4. Most times (much more than half the time)

5. Almost always or always

C. *During sexual intercourse, how often are you able to maintain your erection after you have penetrated (entered) your partner?*

0. Did not attempt intercourse

1. Almost never or never

2. A few times (much less than half the time)

3. Sometimes (about half the time)

4. Most times (much more than half the time)

5. Almost always or always

D. *During sexual intercourse, how difficult is it to maintain your erection to completion and orgasm?*

    0. Did not attempt intercourse

    1. Extremely difficult

    2. Very difficult

    3. Difficult

    4. Slightly difficult

    5. Not difficult

E. *When you attempt sexual intercourse, how often is it satisfactory for you?*

    0. Did not attempt intercourse

    1. Almost never or never

    2. A few times (much less than half the time)

    3. Sometimes (about half the time)

    4. Most times (much more than half the time)

    5. Almost always or always

Add up your score. If your total is less than 21, you may have ED. Make an appointment to meet with your health professional to discuss these issues and possible treatment options.

If you have ED but don't voice your concern, the issue can develop into an overwhelming problem within your relationship. You may feel that it comments negatively on your masculinity, and your partner may feel that it represents your view of her attractiveness and commitment to the relationship. Although you may see it as an embarrassing issue, don't avoid it.

Have you discussed this issue with anyone yet? Have you shared it with your partner? Successful treatment starts with an important first step: you must tell someone. Ask for help and don't give up until you find the treatment that works for you. An experienced health professional can offer effective treatment options. In addition to sharing details about your problem, you will need to provide a detailed medical history and take several blood tests to examine different hormone levels.

Dave finally visited his doctor and had a very productive session. His physician adjusted his medication dose, which improved his blood sugar levels. He also started taking Viagra, one of several medications now available to treat ED. This enabled him to maintain an erection much more often than before. Both he and Laura are relieved—and a lot more satisfied.

Here are suggestions to help make it easier for you and your partner to discuss ED:

1. Find a quiet, stress-free time to begin the discussion. It may be best to speak about it away from the bedroom.

2. Ask for support. Some treatments require lovemaking to be planned ahead to allow medication to take effect. Your partner's cooperation is important to the success of any treatment that you choose.

3. Don't bring up unrelated issues. This is a medical problem. There is no need to allow the discussion to deteriorate into a fault-finding session. Focus on plans for the future, not bad feelings from the past.

4. If it seems appropriate, use touch as a way to connect during your discussion. Handholding and hugging can be a comforting affirmation of your commitment to each other.

Causes of Erectile Dysfunction

Diabetes is only one of the many causes of ED. Others include:

- Blood vessel or vascular disease

- Cancer treatments

- Neurologic conditions

- Medications

- Surgery, especially for prostate problems

- Excessive smoking and alcohol use

- Testosterone deficiency

- Depression

- Emotional issues, such as lack of interest in a partner due to weight gain, boredom, tension in the relationship, or other personal issues

Regardless of the cause, ED usually can be treated successfully. The following are several often successful treatment options.

Viagra and Beyond

Viagra (Sidenafil), first on the block to treat ED, has been joined by two additional choices, Levitra (Vardenafil) and Cialis (Tadalafil). All improve ED in men with diabetes, are well-tolerated, and have few side effects. Because they increase and maintain blood flow to the penis, they cannot be taken with medicines such as vasodilators and nitrates (used to treat angina or chest pain) that have a similar action. Speak with your physician to see if any are appropriate for you.

All three of these treatments have raised public awareness of this common and uncomfortable topic. These drugs work by increasing the body's nitric oxide levels, a substance that helps the penis fill with blood and develop a successful erection. A dose is taken prior to intercourse and requires sexual stimulation to produce results.

Over the past few years, more than 10 million men have enjoyed the benefits of Viagra. Steve, one of our authors, recalls a patient's recent experience with it:

> I had a patient with type 1 diabetes who recently told me that Viagra did not work for him. He said that after he took the medication, he sat on the couch and read a book about growing tomatoes! You must have sexual stimulation for Viagra to work effectively.

Levitra is another medication that works well in men with diabetes. Both Levitra and Viagra should be taken approximately one hour prior to intimate activity to allow adequate time to be spontaneous and romantic. Like Viagra, Levitra requires sexual stimulation for a successful erection.

Cialis can be taken up to 36 hours prior to intimate activity. This lets you and your partner enjoy your time together at a natural and relaxed pace. It takes effect within 30 minutes and remains active for up to 36 hours (plenty of time for sex and growing tomatoes!). The manufacturer encourages users to avoid excessive alcohol intake, defined as five glasses of wine or five shots of whiskey. In France, Cialis is called "Le Weekend" because of its long-lasting effect. One pill taken at a hearty lunch on Friday is rumored to be all one needs to stay sexually active for an entire weekend.

Possible side effects from these medications include headache, nasal congestion, or upset stomach. Viagra and Levitra may induce a temporary blue tint in your vision that

can last for several hours, but it is not permanent or dangerous. These problems diminish with continued use.

Penile Injections

This treatment sounds like a form of torture but actually works quite well. You inject a specially prepared medication, such as Alprostadil, directly into the penis with a convenient autoinjector. The medicine relaxes the penile tissues
and helps an erection develop in a way that is similar to
Viagra, Cialis, and Levitra but has a higher success rate since
it enters the penis directly. An erection occurs within 5–20
minutes and is usually enhanced by sexual stimulation. For
most individuals, the effects last less than an hour. Injections
should only be given once every 24 hours and not more often than three times a week. Sticking a needle directly into
the penis may not sound appealing, but with few nerve end-
ings at the injection site, any discomfort is minimal.

Penile Suppositories

Instead of injecting Alprostadil, a suppository can be
inserted into the penis. It works in the same way as a penile
injection but does not have as high a success rate.

Hormone Therapy

Patients with a testosterone deficiency can be easily
treated with hormonal replacement therapy, either by injection
or skin patches. A simple non-fasting blood test checks for testosterone deficiency. Men on this type of therapy should be
carefully screened for prostate cancer by taking regular blood
tests for prostate-specific antigen (PSA) and by digital rectal
examinations. Low testosterone is an uncommon cause of ED
and only occurs in about 5 percent of all cases.

Vacuum Constrictor Devices

Mechanical devices are helpful and work best with a partner you know well, since they take some of the spontaneity out of sex and require understanding and support. A vacuum constrictor is a great option for men with diabetes. The device's plastic chamber is placed over the penis. A vacuum pump creates negative pressure within the chamber and enables the penis to fill with blood. Once engorged, a thick rubber band-like ring is placed over the base of the penis to help hold the erection long enough for intercourse. No surgery or injection is required.

Constriction rings can also be used alone, without a vacuum device. They are ideal for men who are able to achieve, but can't maintain an erection. Known as venous flow constrictors, these rings are found in pharmacies or shops that specialize in sexual enhancement items.

Surgical Solutions

Surgical implants range from semi-rigid to inflatable and use pumps to inflate and deflate the penis as desired. Surgical complications are low, especially when the patient's diabetes control is stable prior to surgery. The internal anatomy of the penis changes with the implantation of these devices, which makes other options ineffective if the implant ever needs to be removed. Surgery is normally considered only after more conservative measures have been tried.

Lifestyle Approaches to ED

1. Exercise

Regular exercise improves circulation, energizes you, and can improve your mood—all important for sexual health. In addition to these benefits, exercise enhances insulin sensitivity, improves cardiovascular risk factors such as blood pressure and lipid levels, can reduce your need for diabetes medications, and helps you meet your weight-loss goals. Choose a variety of activities to do daily or several times each week.

2. Stop Smoking

Although smoking is a very difficult habit to stop, it's worthwhile to try because smoking can affect your sexual performance. Many treatment options, ranging from medications to support groups, can help you break the habit. If you are ready to quit, discuss the different smoking cessation options with your diabetes care giver. Although smoking cessation is not the most powerful ED remedy, many men see dramatic improvement in their ED after quitting.

3. Limit Alcohol Intake

Too much alcohol can make it difficult to get or maintain an erection, whether you have diabetes or not. Moderation is the key. Consume your alcoholic beverages with food to help prevent a low blood sugar reaction. Remember, alcoholic drinks have calories and can promote unwanted weight gain. If you do imbibe, regardless of the amount, test your blood sugar frequently so that you can treat both high and low levels.

Women Have Issues Too

Women with diabetes can also experience sexual challenges that affect a couple's sexual enjoyment.

1. Do you experience lubrication problems during sexual activity?

2. Do you have a decreased interest in sexual activity?

3. Are you having difficulty achieving orgasm?

4. Do you have pain during intercourse?

5. Do you have a loss of sensation in the vaginal area?

If you answered yes to any of the above questions, you may have sexual difficulties related to your diabetes. Lubrication problems can cause discomfort during intercourse. A decrease in sexual interest or reduced ability to achieve orgasm will make intimacy far less enjoyable. Pain during intimate activity may be caused by a variety of problems including urinary tract infection or yeast infection, both common in women who have diabetes. A loss of sensation may also be related. As with ED, good diabetes control can improve these problems or help avoid them altogether. Share your concerns with your partner and health professional.

Susan and Tom were both frustrated. Lately, intercourse had become so uncomfortable for Susan, who has had type 2 diabetes for about three years, that she dreaded each time Tom came close. They discussed the problem, but all Tom could suggest were different sexual positions that he found in a book. She recalled reading about lubrication problems in a woman's magazine but couldn't remember the suggested causes or remedies. Neither Susan nor Tom had any idea that Susan's diabetes was the major factor keeping her from enjoying their intimate moments to the fullest.

Susan visited her doctor, who performed a complete physical to search for possible causes. Her A1C, the measure of blood sugar control over the past three months, was 11.0 percent, significantly higher than her goal of 6.5–7.0 percent. Both agreed that her chronically high blood sugar levels could be a cause.

Susan's doctor increased her oral diabetes medication and suggested vaginal lubricants for the dryness. She also met with a registered dietitian to improve her food choices. As a result of these steps, Susan's A1C dropped to 8.0 percent and her sexual interest improved. Susan and Tom were pleased with the results.

Lubrication and Arousal Problems

The body depends on its nervous and circulatory systems to initiate vaginal lubrication. High blood glucose levels can, over an extended period of time, lead to nerve damage that not only reduces these secretions but also lowers sensitivity. Without adequate lubrication, irritation and pain may occur during sexual activity and make intimacy extremely unpleasant.

Water-based, water-soluble vaginal lubricants, such as K-Y jelly and Astroglide, are available at local pharmacies. They help encourage sexual arousal and increase comfort during intercourse. Hand creams, body lotions and petroleum-based lubricants, such as Vaseline, can cause further irritation and should be avoided.

Orgasm

An orgasm is one of the many pleasurable physical responses that a woman has during sexual activity. A lack of desire, vaginal dryness, nerve damage, and abnormal blood glucose levels all interfere with a woman's ability to achieve an orgasm. This problem can be frustrating for a couple. Fortunately, you can improve this situation:

1. *Normalize your blood sugar levels before becoming intimate.* Some women report that they can't achieve an orgasm when their blood glucose levels are poorly controlled. Aim to maintain your A1C level within a healthy range (below 6.5–7.0 percent).

2. *Use a lubricant.* Vaginal lubricants safely add moisture to the genital area as mentioned above. Introduce lubricants into your bedroom activities. They can enhance your time together without being a reminder of any sexual problem.

"I always think it is worth it to have a tube of Astroglide on your nightstand, as it implies you have a very exciting life," says Dr. Susan Love, author of *Dr. Susan Love's Breast Book* and *Dr. Susan Love's Menopause and Hormone Book* and a founder of the breast cancer advocacy movement. (Dr. Susan Love's website is: www.susanlovemd.org)

3. *Focus on your body.* Do you feel unattractive? If you are unhappy with your weight, create a weight-loss plan with the help of a registered dietitian. If you feel depressed or uncomfortable about sex, see a mental health professional who can help you work through these feelings.

4. *Reduce stress.* If your relationship is stressful, try to talk out your problems. If necessary, meet with a counselor who can help you get your romantic life back on track. Do some form of physical activity each day, have a massage, listen to soothing music, read a book, or take a leisurely walk. Don't underestimate the relaxing power of these types of activities.

The stresses of daily life can interfere with intimate moments. The last thing that should be on your mind while in the bedroom is your list of pressing household and business errands. You don't have to be superwoman. If you feel overwhelmed by everything on your plate, drop some of your activities. Your children do not have to participate in every available activity known to man and you don't have to volunteer at every event. Here is what Janis, one of our authors, suggests:

I always volunteered an enormous amount. When my activities became so time consuming that they created tension between me and my husband, I adjusted my priorities. Now, I no longer help in areas that others can do equally as well, such as stuffing envelopes or collecting money at events. If I can add my special touch to something I am passionate about, then I'll volunteer. I choose my outside activities carefully and schedule time for myself. I exercise each day and spend time with friends. When I am good to myself, I am much more relaxed and better able to enjoy my marriage and family.

Vaginal Infections

Yeast and urinary tract infections often develop in women with diabetes and cause a couple's intimate life to be put on hold.

Vaginal yeast infections develop when the normal balance of vaginal organisms changes and encourages an overgrowth of yeast cells. This happens for a variety of reasons, including diabetes. Common symptoms are:

- Vaginal itching

- Irritated skin in the genital area

- A white vaginal discharge with an odorless cottage cheese-like appearance

- Burning or pain in the genital area during sexual intercourse

- Discomfort in the genital area while urinating

Urinary tract infections (UTI) are rarely serious but need to be treated promptly. The urinary tract includes several organs that perform different functions. The kidneys produce urine, the bladder stores it, the ureters transport it from the kidneys to the bladder, and the urethra carries the urine from the bladder to the outside of the body. Most infections affect the bladder or the kidneys. Symptoms of UTI include:

- Pain or burning when urinating

- A frequent urge to urinate small amounts

- A tender or heavy feeling in the lower abdomen

- Cloudy or unpleasant-smelling urine

- Pain on one side of your back beneath the rib cage

- Fever, chills, nausea, and vomiting

Treatment of Vaginal Infections

If this is the first time that you have had a vaginal infection, see your health professional to confirm your suspicions. He or she may suggest a vaginal exam and test your urine or any discharge to be certain of the diagnosis. Oral antibiotics will help cure a UTI, and over-the-counter medications can treat yeast infections.

Here are a few other treatment suggestions:

1. Maintain your blood glucose levels as close to your target range as possible. High levels encourage the growth of unwanted bacteria.

2. Avoid tight underwear, pantyhose, pants, or shorts that restrict the flow of air.

3. Wear all-cotton underwear.

4. Drink artificially sweetened cranberry juice to help treat and prevent urinary tract infections.

5. Eat a daily serving of low-fat yogurt. Be sure that it contains active cultures. It may help prevent future vaginal infections.

6. Wipe from the front to the back after using the toilet to avoid contaminating the vaginal area with any bacteria from the rectal region.

7. Bathe regularly to keep the vaginal area clean.

8. Drink plenty of water.

9. Empty your bladder every two hours while awake.

10. Your partner should shower prior to intercourse to be sure that he is clean and will not introduce harmful bacteria into your vaginal area.

Don't let diabetes or any other problem rob you of sexual fulfillment. Be open about your sexual difficulties. Discuss them with your partner and a trusted healthcare professional.

Other Issues That Affect Your Sex Life

Waning Interest

For both women and men, sexual interest usually involves a combination of both physical and psychological factors. If you have abnormal blood glucose levels, feel depressed or fatigued, or have become bored or dissatisfied with your relationship, it is difficult to feel sexual. Antidepressants, high blood pressure medicines, and other medications can affect your interest in being intimate. If you believe that you are less attractive because of unwanted weight gain, dry skin, rashes, or marks from injections and pump infusion sets, you may feel uncomfortable interacting sexually with your loved one.

Discuss your concerns with your partner, and, if needed, meet with a mental health professional to help you deal with them. A lack of sexual interest is not a permanent casualty of diabetes. If you feel awkward about your appearance, turn down the lights and add the glow of candlelight and soft music to your lovemaking area. Invest in flattering sleepwear, perfumes, and colognes. You will feel attractive and your partner will hopefully appreciate the added visual and sensual stimulation.

Enjoy sex! There's no need for your diabetes to get in the way. If you're self-conscious, have sex in the dark.

—Aimée

Bad Breath

Is your breath "kissably sweet"? If not, it could be from your diabetes. Everyone, with or without diabetes, must take care of their dental health. But individuals with diabetes are more prone to develop periodontal disease, a painless disease of the supporting tissues of the teeth, gums, and bones of the mouth that can affect your breath and cause serious health problems.

- Do your gums bleed easily when brushing or flossing?
- Do you have loose teeth?
- Are your gums red, swollen, or tender?
- Do you have tartar on your teeth (creamy, brown, hard masses on the tooth's surface)?
- Do you notice a change in how your teeth fit together when you bite?
- Do you have pain chewing?
- Are your teeth sensitive?

If you answered yes to any of these questions, you may have periodontal disease. See your dentist for a complete evaluation. Have your teeth professionally cleaned at least twice a year, floss daily, and use a mouthwash that does not contain alcohol, which dries out your gums. Hydrogen peroxide half diluted with water is an effective and inexpensive mouthwash alternative.

Very high glucose levels over several days can also affect your breath, especially if your body begins using fat, rather than glucose, as its energy source. The ketone bodies produced during fat breakdown often create an unpleasant breath odor. Keep your sugar level within your target range to reduce or eliminate this problem.

Tips for Successful Intimacy

Sweets for the Sweet: Hypoglycemia in the Bedroom

A drop in blood glucose levels during sexual activity can put the brakes on a romantic evening.

> Jan and Kevin were starting to get romantic when Jan noticed that Kevin was uncharacteristically losing interest. His movement became slowed and he just lay there. His skin was getting moist and clammy. Jan ran for his blood sugar monitor. Kevin checked his sugar and it was in the low 50s. Fortunately he had orange juice boxes at the bedside and he quickly treated his low. Kevin now checks before things get heavy.

To prevent blood glucose lows during sexual activity, test your blood sugars before getting intimate, if possible. If your blood glucose levels are below 70mg/dl (or low as defined by your physician), follow the "15 Rule," described in Chapter 6, to return your levels to your target range.

Sex and an Insulin Pump

> There's no norm in sex. Norm is the name of a guy who lives in Brooklyn.
> —Dr. Alex Comfort, author of *The Joy of Sex*,
> (Crown Publishers)

There are two options with the insulin pump: wear it or disconnect it. A pump can be safely removed for about 45 minutes to an hour if you use Humalog or Novolog insulin. Some people leave their pump on when the spontaneity of the moment takes over.

> I keep my pump on about 90 percent of the time and un-hook it quickly if it gets in the way. Once, afterward, I went into the bathroom, and it fell into the toilet. Now *that* was funny! To truly enjoy sex with a pump, don't give it a lot of attention. Your pump should not inhibit any part of your life; it's meant to make life easier.
>
> —Aimée

If your pump gets disconnected during sexual activity, reconnect when done. Test your blood glucose and take a correction dose of insulin if needed.

Here are some tips for nurturing intimacy:

1. If you have sexual difficulties, attend counseling sessions as a couple if you can. This will help both partners be active participants in any treatment that the therapist suggests.

2. If your partner attempts to quit smoking, it may alter your social life in the short run. He or she may temporarily need to stay away from the smoking temptations of nightclubs and other social gatherings. Together, search for alternate forms of entertainment, like movies and plays. If you both smoke, try to cut back or quit together.

3. Be patient and supportive when sexual difficulties occur.

4. Be open about your sexual needs. It is upsetting if you can't meet the sexual needs of the one you love.

Experiment with sexual positions and allow time for additional stimulation. Encourage discussion with a member of your partner's healthcare team if the two of you cannot resolve an issue.

5. Don't panic if the pump is accidentally pulled out during sexual activity. You will not be injured. Even if some bleeding occurs, it is not harmful.

6. Exercise together. It is fun and will enhance your relationship as you both improve your health.

7. Has your spouse's physical appearance become a sexual "turnoff"? Reconnect on a non-sexual level by taking walks and enjoying weekly outings. Rediscover the person you love.

Don't Let Diabetes Block Romance

Here is a checklist to help you keep diabetes *out* of the bedroom:

✔ Blood glucose monitor
Check before lovemaking begins. Sex, like other forms of physical activity, can induce hypoglycemia (low blood glucose). Treat abnormal blood sugar levels as directed by your healthcare team.

✔ Snacks
In case of unexpected low blood sugar, keep fast-acting carbohydrate snacks close by, such as glucose tablets or juice boxes.

✔ Alcoholic beverages
Remember, everything in moderation. One to two drinks is a safe limit, but know your personal limits. Some individuals tolerate more, some less. Consume alcoholic bever-

ages in moderation with food or a meal, and test your glucose level frequently.

✔ Alcohol-free creams and oils

Alcohol dries the skin and promotes cracking, so don't use products that contain it. If you rub on scented and flavored oils, avoid areas with skin folds such as armpits, the groin area, between the toes, and under the breasts. When moist, these areas can encourage the development of fungal and bacterial infections.

✔ Hot tub

A brief dip with a loving partner is a relaxing and sensual experience. If you have a loss of sensation in your feet and legs, check the temperature of the tub before entering. Enjoy your time in the tub if it relaxes you and puts you in the mood. If you have heart disease and stay in a whirlpool bath for over 20–30 minutes, it may cause your blood pressure to drop too low. Dry your skin thoroughly after exiting the tub; excess moisture encourages the growth of bacteria that cause infections.

✔ Bathtub or shower

Like the hot tub, a bubble bath or shower is a terrific way to relax and begin a wonderful evening of sexual activity. But keep your bath brief. Soaking in a tub for hours is not recommended for individuals with diabetes as it tends to soften and dry out the skin, leaving it susceptible to bacterial growth.

WHAT A WOMAN MAY WANT A MAN TO KNOW ABOUT SEXUAL ISSUES

1. Emotions play a great role in my ability to get "in the mood." My sexual interest can be enhanced by romantic gifts, tender touches, and words of love and affection.

2. When I don't feel well, it is difficult to enjoy sexual activities.

3. I may find it awkward to discuss sexual issues. Often times, I may be uncertain about what to ask of you. Please be patient and supportive.

WHAT A MAN MAY WANT A WOMAN TO KNOW ABOUT SEXUAL ISSUES

1. ED has nothing to do with how attractive or desirable you are.

2. An erection problem is devastating to the male ego. I feel terrible when this happens and really need your support.

3. I may have difficulty being open about such personal issues. Even if I do not discuss them with you, I do appreciate your love and concern.

Don't let diabetes intrude on your most private moments. You deserve to have fulfilling intimate relationships. Discuss any sexual problems with a trusted healthcare professional who can help you find solutions that will work for you.

Suggested Resources

ORGANIZATIONS

American Association of Diabetes Educators (AADE)
The American Association of Diabetes Educators is a multi-disciplinary professional membership organization dedicated to advancing the practice of diabetes self-management training and care as integral components of healthcare for persons with diabetes, and lifestyle management for the prevention of diabetes.

American Association of Diabetes Educators
100 W. Monroe Street, Suite 400
Chicago, IL 60603
Phone:1-800-338-3633
E-mail: aade@aadenet.org
Website: www.diabeteseducator.org

American Diabetes Association (ADA)
The American Diabetes Association is the nation's leading non-profit health organization providing diabetes research, information, and advocacy. Its mission is to prevent and cure diabetes and to improve the lives of all people affected by diabetes.

American Diabetes Association
ATTN: National Call Center
1701 North Beauregard Street
Alexandria, VA 22311
Phone: 1-800-DIABETES (1-800-342-2383)
E-mail: askada@diabetes.org
Website: www.diabetes.org

American Heart Association (AHA)
   The American Heart Association is a national voluntary health
   agency whose mission is to reduce disability and death from
   cardiovascular diseases and stroke.

American Heart Association
National Center
7272 Greenville Avenue
Dallas, TX 75231
Phone: 1-800-AHA-USA1 (1-800-242-8721)
Website: www.americanheart.org

Behavorial Diabetes Institute (BDI)
   The Behavioral Diabetes Institute is dedicated to addressing
   the unmet psychological needs of people with diabetes.

Behavioral Diabetes Institute
PO Box 501866
San Diego, CA 92150-1866
Phone: 858-336-8693
E-mail: info@behavioraldiabetes.org
Website: www.behavioraldiabetes.org

Diabetes Research Institute (DRI)
   The Diabetes Research Institute is an international center
   dedicated exclusively to the cure and treatment of diabetes.

Diabetes Research Institute Foundation
3440 Hollywood Boulevard, Suite 100
Hollywood, FL 33021
Phone: 1-800-321-3437 (954-964-4040)
Fax: 954-964-7036
Website: www.drinet.org

International Diabetes Center (IDC)
   The International Diabetes Center works to ensure that every
   individual with diabetes or at risk for diabetes receives the best
   possible care.

International Diabetes Center
3800 Park Nicollet Boulevard
Minneapolis, Minnesota 55416-2699

Phone: 952-993-3393
Toll-free:1-888-825-6315
Fax: 952-993-1302
E-mail: idcdiabetes@parknicollet.com
Website: www.parknicollet.com/diabetes

Joslin Diabetes Center (JDC)
Joslin is a nonprofit organization dedicated to finding a cure for diabetes and improving the lives of people with diabetes.

Joslin Diabetes Center
1 Joslin Place
Boston, MA 02215
Phone: 617-732-2400
Website: www.joslin.org

Juvenile Diabetes Research Foundation International (JDRFI)
This is the leading charitable funder and advocate of type 1 (juvenile) diabetes research worldwide. Its mission is to find a cure for diabetes and its complications through the support of research.

Juvenile Diabetes Research Foundation International
120 Wall Street
New York, NY 10005-4001
Phone: 1-800-533-CURE (1-800-533-2873)
Fax: 212-785-9595
E-mail: info@jdrf.org
Website: www.jdrf.org

TCOYD—Taking Control of Your Diabetes
TCOYD is a nonprofit organization dedicated to educating and motivating people with diabetes and their loved ones to take an active role in their condition in order to live healthier and happier lives.

TCOYD—Taking Control of Your Diabetes
1110 Camino Del Mar, Suite B
Del Mar, CA 92014
Phone: 858-755-5683 (toll-free: 1-800-99-TCOYD)
Fax: 858-755-6854
Website: www.tcoyd.org

BOOKS FROM SURREY

Website: www.surreybooks.com

Diabetes Snacks, Treats, and Easy Eats by Barbara Grunes

Eat Out, Eat Right! by Hope S. Warshaw, MMSc, RD, CDE

Light & Easy Diabetes Cuisine by Betty Marks

1,001 Delicious Recipes for People with Diabetes, edited by Linda Eugene, RD, CDE; Sue Spitler; and Linda R. Yoakam, RD, MS

BOOKS

ADA Complete Guide to Diabetes, 3rd edition, American Diabetes Association (ADA, 2003).
Available at: 1-800-DIABETES, www.diabetes.org, Amazon.com, Barnes & Noble.com

Charting a Course to Wellness: Creative Ways of Living with Heart Disease, Treena and Graham Kerr (ADA, 2004).
Available at:1-800-DIABETES, www.grahamkerr.com, www.diabetes.org, Amazon.com, Barnes & Noble.com

Complete Guide to Carb Counting, 2nd edition, Hope S. Warshaw, MMSc, RD, CDE, and Karmeen Kulkarni, MS, RD, CDE (ADA, 2004).
Available at:1-800-DIABETES, www.hopewarshaw.com, www.diabetes.org, Amazon.com, Barnes & Noble.com, and major bookstores

Diabetes Burnout: What to Do When You Can't Take It Anymore, William H. Polonsky, PhD, CDE (ADA, 1999). Also available in audiocassette.
Available at: 1-800-DIABETES, www.diabetes.org, Amazon.com, Barnes & Noble.com

Diabetes for Dummies, Alan L. Rubin, MD (John Wiley & Sons, 1999).
Available at: Amazon.com, Barnes & Noble.com

The Diabetes Problem Solver: Quick Answers to Your Questions about Treatment and Self-Care, Nancy Touchette, PhD (ADA, 1999).
Available at: 1-800-DIABETES, www.diabetes.org, Amazon.com

The Diabetic Athlete: Prescriptions for Exercise and Sports, Shari Colberg, PhD (Human Kinetics, 2000).
Available at: Amazon.com, Barnes & Noble.com

A Field Guide to Type 1 Diabetes, American Diabetes Association (ADA, 2002).
Available at: 1-800-DIABETES, www.diabetes.org, Amazon.com, Barnes & Noble.com

A Field Guide to Type 2 Diabetes, American Diabetes Association (ADA, 2004).
Available at: 1-800-DIABETES, www.diabetes.org, Amazon.com, Barnes & Noble.com

For Each Other: Sharing Sexual Intimacy, revised edition, Lonnie Barbach, PhD (Signet, 2000).
Available at Amazon.com, Barnes & Noble.com

For Yourself: The Fulfillment of Female Sexuality, reissue edition, Lonnie Barbach, PhD (Signet, 2001).
Available at Amazon.com, Barnes & Noble.com

Making Love the Way We Used To, Or Better: Secrets to Satisfying Midlife Sexuality, Alan M. Altman, MD, and Laurie Ashner (McGraw-Hill/Contemporary Books, 2002).
Available at Amazon.com, Barnes & Noble.com

The New Male Sexuality, revised edition, Bernie Zilbergeld, PhD (Bantam, 1999).
Available at: Amazon.com, Barnes & Noble.com

Psyching Out Diabetes: A Postive Approach to Your Negative Emotions, revised 3rd edition, Richard Rubin, PhD, CDE (Lowell House, 1999).
Available at: Amazon.com, Barnes & Noble.com

101 Tips for Coping with Diabetes, American Diabetes Association
(ADA, 2003).
Available at: 1-800-DIABETES, www.diabetes.org, Amazon.com,
Barnes & Noble.com

Smart Pumping: A Practical Approach to the Insulin Pump,
Howard Wolpert, MD (ADA, 2002).
Available at: 1-800-DIABETES, www.diabetes.org, Amazon.com,
Barnes & Noble.com

Taking Control of Your Diabetes, 2nd edition, Steven V. Edelman,
MD (Professional Communications, Inc., 2001).
Available at: TCOYD.org, Amazon.com, Barnes & Noble.com

The Uncomplicated Guide to Diabetes Complications, 2nd edition,
Marvin E. Levin, MD, and Michael A. Pfeifer, MD, MS, CDE,
FACE (ADA, 2002).
Available at: 1-800-DIABETES, www.diabetes.org, Amazon.com,
Barnes & Noble.com

MAGAZINES

Diabetes Forecast
This is the official magazine of the American Diabetes Association.
It comes free with membership in the ADA. Call   1-800-DIA-
BETES or visit www.diabetes.org to join.

Diabetes Health
Formerly known as Diabetes Interview magazine, this publication
is available on the magazine racks of many major booksellers. Call
1-800-488-8468 for subscription information.

Diabetes Positive!
This publication is given out free by health professionals. Ask your
diabetes educator about it or call 770-576-1938 for subscription
information.

Diabetes Self-Management
This bimonthly publication is commonly seen in healthcare
waiting rooms. Call 1-800-234-0923 to subscribe.

WEBSITES

www.behavioraldiabetes.org
The official website of the Behavioral Diabetes Institute, the world's first organization dedicated to addressing the unmet psychological needs of people with diabetes. It was founded by William H. Polonsky, PhD, CDE, one of our authors.

www.diabetes.org
The official website of the American Diabetes Association.

www.parknicollet.com/diabetes
The official website of the International Diabetes Center.

www.drinet.org
The official website of the diabetes Research Institute.

www.americanheart.org
The official website of the American Heart Association.

www.consumerlab.com
Contains reliable and independent test results of herbal, vitamin, and nutritional supplements.

www.diabeteseducator.org
The official website of the American Association of Diabetes Educators. It can help you locate a qualified educator in your area.

www.diabetic.com
This diabetes product sales site is the home of an excellent diabetes bulletin board monitored by one of our authors, Janis Roszler, RD, CDE, LD/N.

www.medlineplus.com
A service of the U.S. National Library of Medicine and the National Institutes of Health. It contains a wealth of information, including details about different medications—why they are prescribed, how they should be used, special precautions, side effects, and storage information.

www.jdrf.org
The official website of the Juvenile Diabetes Research Foundation.
An excellent source for research updates.

www.joslin.org
The official website of the Joslin Diabetes Center, affiliated with
Harvard University.

www.niddk.nih.gov
National Institute of Diabetes & Digestive & Kidney Diseases
website.

www.mendosa.com
David Mendosa is a freelance medical writer and consultant,
specializing in diabetes. As a hobby, he runs this comprehensive
site that links to an impressive number of diabetes resources and
websites.

www.quackwatch.com
Debunks medical myths. If you read advice on the Internet that
seems too good to be true, check it out here.

www.TCOYD.org
Taking Control of Your Diabetes—this is the official site of the
organization founded by Dr. Steven Edelman, one of our authors.
TCOYD sponsors numerous diabetes seminars throughout the
United States. Check out the upcoming schedule and learn more
about this excellent organization.

www.urbanlegends.about.com
Collects and analyzes Internet urban legends. If you read something that seems unbelievable, verify it here.

www.webmd.com
A reliable source of medical information on any topic.

Index